Urinary Continence

Assessment and Promotion

Mary H. Palmer, PhD, RN, C, FAAN
Senior Staff Fellow
National Institute of Nursing Research
Bethesda, Maryland
Adjunct Associate Professor
Johns Hopkins University School of Nursing
Baltimore, Maryland

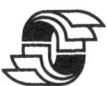

An Aspen Publication®
Aspen Publishers, Inc.
Gaithersburg, Maryland
1996

Library of Congress Cataloging-in-Publication Data

Palmer, Mary H.
Urinary continence: assessment and promotion / Mary H. Palmer.
p. cm.
Rev. ed. of: Urinary incontinence. c1985.
Includes bibliographical references and index.
ISBN 0-8342-0747-8
1. Urinary incontinence—Nursing.
2. Urinary incontinence in old age—Nursing.
I. Palmer, Mary H. Urinary incontinence.
II. Title.
[DNLM: 1. Urinary Incontinence—nursing.
2. Urinary Incontinence—in old age.
WY 164 P175uc 1996]
RC921.I5P35 1996
616.6'2—dc20
DNLM/DLC
for Library of Congress
95-53082
CIP

Copyright © 1996 by Aspen Publishers, Inc.
All rights reserved.

Aspen Publishers, Inc., grants permission for photocopying for limited personal or internal use. This consent does not extend to other kinds of copying, such as copying for general distribution, for advertising or promotional purposes, for creating new collective works, or for resale. For information, address Aspen Publishers, Inc., Permissions Department, 200 Orchard Ridge Drive, Suite 200, Gaithersburg, Maryland 20878.

> The authors have made every effort to ensure the accuracy of the information herein. However, appropriate information sources should be consulted, especially for new or unfamiliar drugs or procedures. It is the responsibility of every practitioner to evaluate the appropriateness of a particular opinion in the context of actual clinical situations and with due consideration to new developments. The authors acknowledge the mention of specific products as examples of products in current clinical practice; however, this should not be construed as endorsements of the products. The authors, editors, and the publisher cannot be held responsible for any typographical or other errors found in this book.

Editorial Resources: Jane Colilla

Library of Congress Catalog Card Number: 95-53082
ISBN: 0-8342-0747-8

Printed in the United States of America

1 2 3 4 5

*To Mildred Holland, RN,
the nurse who taught me the essence of nursing
is Tender Loving Care.*

Table of Contents

Preface	ix
Introduction	xi
Chapter 1—Normal Micturition	**1**
Overview	1
Kidneys and Ureters	1
Bladder and Urethra	1
Spinal Cord	6
Cortical Center of Control	8
Cycle of Normal Micturition	8
Effects of Age	10
Chapter 2—Definitions	**13**
Overview	13
Definitions for Urinary Incontinence	14
Patterns of Incontinence	22
Chapter 3—Associated Factors and Causes	**24**
Prevalence of Incontinence	24
Pathophysiology of Incontinence	29
Causes of Transient Incontinence	30
Urogenital Causes and Factors	31
Neurological Causes	35

Environmental Factors	40
Conclusion	44

Chapter 4—Assessment **47**

Nursing's Role	47
Assessment in the Long-Term Care Setting	51
Assessment of Noninstitutionalized Older Adults	56
Assessment in the Acute Care Setting	62
Voiding Record	62
Conclusion	76

Chapter 5—Treatment **79**

General Guidelines	79
Behavioral Treatment	87
Surgical Interventions	95
Pharmacological Interventions	96
Voiding Maneuvers	100
Treatment of Functional Incontinence	101
Treatment of Transient Incontinence	102
Treatment Settings	104
Conclusion	108

Chapter 6—Psychological Impact **111**

Overview	111
Historical Perspective	111
Psychological Impact on the Older Adult	114
Psychological Impact on the Families	118
Psychological Impact on the Nursing Staff	119
Conclusion	120

Chapter 7—Nursing Care of Incontinent Older Adults **123**

Nursing Role in the Care of Incontinent Older Adults	125
Nursing Care of Incontinent Older Adults	130
How To Set Up a Continence Program	152
Conclusion	157

Chapter 8—Supportive Devices for Urine Control **161**

    Overview 161
    Disposable Absorbent Products 163
    Reusable Briefs and Products 164
    Absorbent Bed Protectors 166
    Absorbent Disposable Bed Protectors 166
    Environmental Modifications 166
    Bedside Commodes 168
    Urinals for Men 168
    Urinals for Women 168
    Bedpans 170
    External Collection Devices for Men 172
    External Collection Devices for Women 173
    Timing Devices 173
    Dampness Detectors 173
    Clothing 174
    Indwelling Catheters 174
    Conclusion 178

Appendix A—Glossary **181**

Appendix B—Additional Sources of Information **190**

Index **193**

Preface

In the past decade, knowledge about the physiology of micturition, the effects of aging, and the causes and factors associated with incontinence has burgeoned. No more is incontinence considered an inevitable consequence of becoming old. Sophisticated assessment techniques and multiple treatment options have replaced palliative care. Continence promotion is gaining pre-eminence as knowledge about the risk factors and causes of incontinence increases. Prevention of incontinence and preservation and restoration of continence are the watchwords in continence care, regardless of the health care setting.

The intent of this book is to serve as a practical guide to continence promotion by increasing knowledge about the risk factors and causes of incontinence, the various treatment options, and nursing strategies in the continence care of older adults. The anticipated audience is nurses, nursing students, and other providers of health care services to older adults.

The objectives of the book are

- to provide the reader with baseline information about normal micturition and the causes and associated factors, assessment, and treatment of urinary incontinence in older adults
- to stimulate discussion among health care providers regarding appropriate interventions to reduce or prevent incontinence and to restore continence
- to dispel the myths that incontinence is inevitable and that treating incontinence is futile
- to promote comprehensive and dignified nursing care that incorporates continence in the philosophy and standards of nursing practice

This book acquaints the reader with the many complex issues surrounding the topics of urinary continence and incontinence. References have been included at the end of each chapter. The reader is encouraged to use this information to gain deeper understanding of specific aspects of urinary incontinence. It is recommended that the reader stay abreast of current research findings and information about technological advances and new resources. This information should be shared with other members of the health care team to promote continence in any setting where health care services are provided. By understanding the causes of urinary incontinence and by using appropriate interventions, nurses and other health care providers may be able to prevent incontinence, relieve the physical and psychological consequences of incontinence, and restore continence.

Introduction

Urinary incontinence has long been thought of as an inevitable consequence of old age. Older adults and their caregivers have had little hope of curing incontinence and have sought only to clean up its aftermath. Recently, I came across a composition I had written in my freshman year of college about my first job as a geriatric nursing assistant. The description of my apprehensions while learning how to shave men, make beds the "right" way, and perform other basic nursing skills made me smile until I came to the following passage: "After lunch the RN in charge asked me if I knew what incontinence meant. I hadn't the slightest idea. She explained as people grow older, they couldn't control their bowels and bladder. It was my job to care for them and to keep them comfortable." The notion that incontinence was an inevitable process of aging persisted for several years until I learned through my clinical experience and readings that incontinence need not be a fixture of old age. Aging alone will not cause incontinence.

These words were part of the Introduction for the first edition of this book published in 1985. That edition, titled *Urinary Incontinence*, reflected the growing awareness among clinicians and researchers that incontinence was a treatable condition and that the quality of life of incontinent older adults could be improved.

With this edition, the new title, *Urinary Continence: Assessment and Promotion*, reflects the new focus on continence. Continence care certainly involves assessment and treatment of incontinence. However, it also involves prevention of incontinence and the restoration of continence by providing information to older adults and caregivers about normal micturition, functioning of the urogenital structures, the effects of age, potential urogenital disruptions, and interventions to promote urogenital functions.

Some of the goals that guide current research efforts and clinical care are the restoration and maintenance of continence; alleviation of the physical, psychological, and social effects of incontinence; and improvement of the quality of life of incontinent adults. There are also intense efforts in the development of comprehensive health promotion interventions to prevent incontinence from ever occurring in people of all ages.

Continence is a complex phenomenon. Research and technological advances are rapidly increasing knowledge. Clinicians are challenged to keep current with these advances and appropriately apply new knowledge and technology in clinical practice. Instead of being ashamed and fearing detection, incontinent older adults should be able to seek help openly from health care providers who are knowledgeable about the condition and who are ready to provide comprehensive assessment and effective treatment that promotes continence.

CHAPTER

1

Normal Micturition

OVERVIEW

Continence is a state in which a person possesses and exercises the ability to store urine and to micturate at a socially acceptable time and place. Micturition is the final step in the elimination of fluid wastes from the body via the urinary tract. Other terms for micturition include urination, voiding, and passing water.

This chapter briefly discusses normal micturition, which is the storage and emptying of urine from the bladder, and the anatomical structures and their functions necessary to achieve this process. The effects of aging on normal micturition are also discussed.

KIDNEYS AND URETERS

The process of urinary elimination begins in the kidneys. The primary functions of the two kidneys are to remove metabolic wastes from the blood and to maintain homeostasis. Each kidney is approximately 11 cm long and is located on the posterior abdominal wall near the lower thoracic vertebrae. Urine is transported from the kidneys to the bladder by the ureters, which are two fibromuscular tubes approximately 40 to 45 cm long. The physiologic rate of urine transport ranges from approximately 20 to 100 ml/hr (Chancellor & Blavais, 1994). The ureters attach to the posterior lateral surfaces of the urinary bladder (see Figure 1–1).

BLADDER AND URETHRA

The main functions of the bladder, which is a sterile vesica, are to store and to empty urine from the body in a coordinated and efficient manner. The bladder is

2   URINARY CONTINENCE

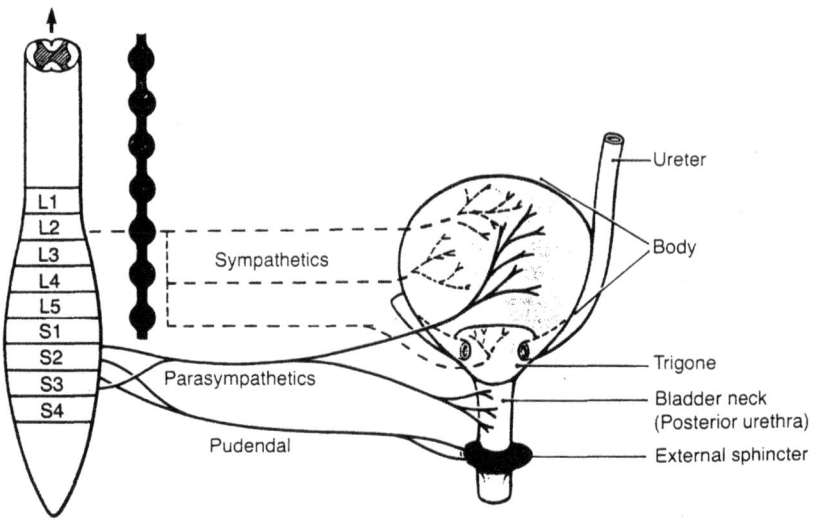

Figure 1–1 The Urinary Bladder and Its Innervation. *Source:* Reprinted from *Basic Neuroscience Anatomy and Physiology*, 2nd ed., by A. Guyton, p. 358, with permission of W.B. Saunders, © 1991.

---

capable of storing approximately 600 to 800 ml of sterile urine, although voluntary voiding usually occurs before this volume is reached (Spence, 1990).

The bladder, a hollow muscular vesica, is composed of two main parts: the body and the neck (see Figure 1–1). The body of the bladder is the major portion of the bladder where urine accumulates. The smooth muscle of the bladder body, the detrusor, is a complex of intermeshing muscle fibers that can contract in a coordinated fashion. Sensory receptors are located in the detrusor walls, which send signals to the sacral reflex center located at S-2 to S-4 (see Figure 1–2). Usually the detrusor can accumulate 250 to 350 ml of urine with little increase in internal pressure. When the detrusor contracts to empty the bladder, pressure inside the bladder can increase as high as 50 cm H_2O (Brocklehurst, 1992).

The neck of the bladder, which is approximately 2 to 3 cm long, forms the base of the bladder. It has a funnel-like configuration and connects to the urethra. In fact, the neck of the bladder is sometimes called the posterior urethra (see Figure 1–1). The neck of the bladder is composed of smooth muscle and elastic tissue. The tone of this muscle keeps the bladder neck and posterior urethra closed and free of urine as the bladder fills (Spence, 1990).

Another important muscle of the bladder is the trigone. It is a triangular shaped muscle extending from above the urethra in the neck of the bladder, up the

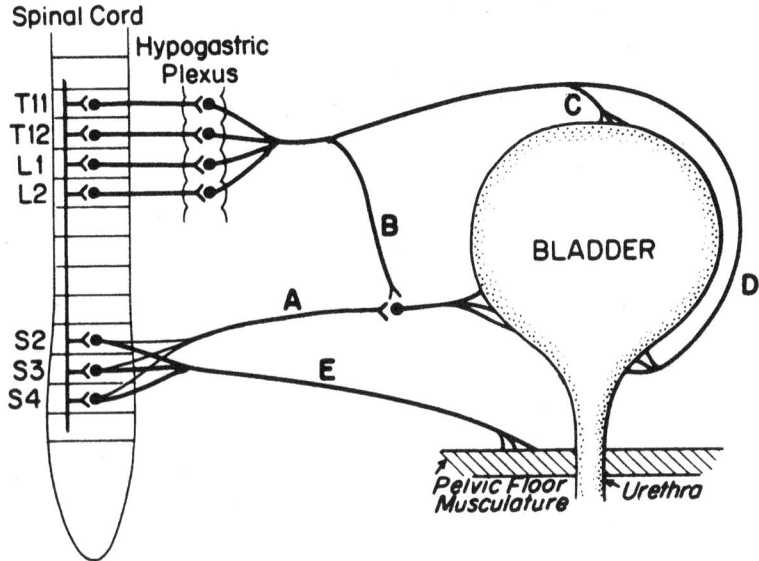

	Type of Nerve	Function
A	PARASYMPATHETIC CHOLINERGIC (Nervi Erigentes)	Bladder contraction
B	SYMPATHETIC	Bladder relaxation (by inhibition of parasympathetic tone)
C	SYMPATHETIC	Bladder relaxation (β adrenergic)
D	SYMPATHETIC	Bladder neck and urethral contraction (α adrenergic)
E	SOMATIC (Pudendal nerve)	Contraction of pelvic floor musculature

Figure 1-2 Peripheral Nerves Involved in Micturition. *Source:* Reprinted from *Essentials of Clinical Geriatrics* 2nd ed., by R. Kane, J. Ouslander and I. Abrass, p. 143, with permission of McGraw-Hill, © 1989.

---

posterior wall of the bladder, and encompassing the ureteral openings (see Figure 1-3) (Guyton, 1991). The trigone performs the important function of applying traction at the ureteral openings during high bladder filling and micturition to prevent reflux of urine back into the ureters (Bradley, 1986). The striated muscle surrounding the external opening of the urethra, sometimes called the external sphincter, can be voluntarily relaxed to facilitate emptying of the bladder.

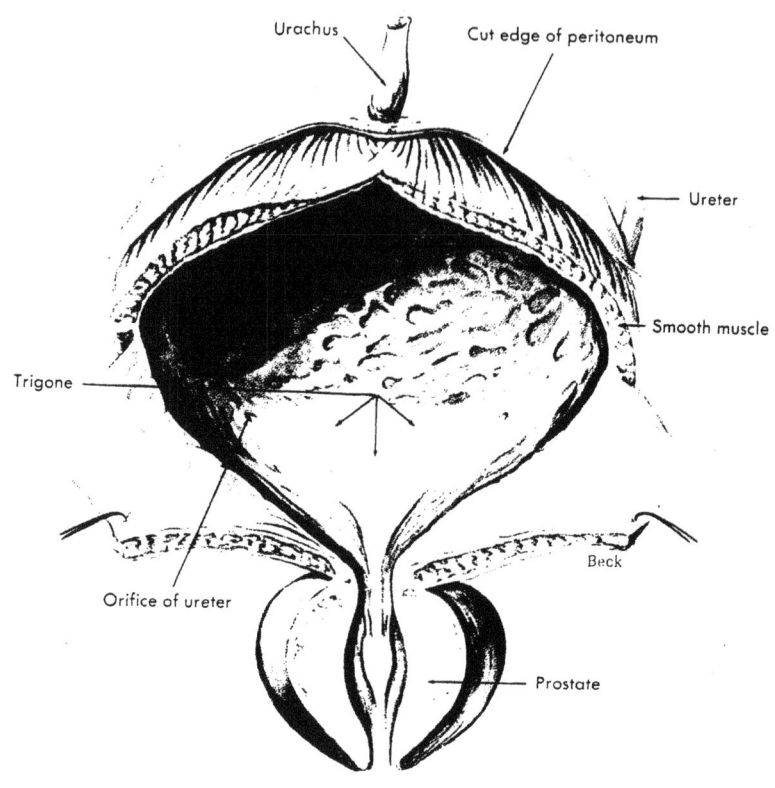

Figure 1–3 The Male Urinary Bladder Cut To Show the Interior. *Source:* Reprinted from *Textbook of Anatomy and Physiology*, 8th ed., by C. Anthony and N. Kolthoff, p. 459, with permission of Mosby-Year Book, © 1971.

The urethra, a muscular tube, is located immediately below the bladder neck and exits the body through the urogenital diaphragm. The area encompassing the urethral, vaginal, and anal openings is often referred to as the pelvic floor. The levator ani muscles provide the structural support to the pelvis and surround the urethra and vagina (Mostwin, 1991). The pubococcygeus is the most important of the three muscles that comprise the levator ani muscle group (Kegel & Powell, 1950).

In women the urethra is short (approximately 4 cm) (see Figure 1–4), whereas in men it is longer (approximately 20 cm) and is surrounded by the prostate gland as it first exits the bladder (see Figure 1–5). The location of the urethra in relation to the levator ani is important, since these muscles support the bladder neck and are in a constant state of contraction (tone) (DeLancy, 1990). The levator ani elevates the bladder neck, helping to form the posterior urethrovesical angle, which is critical to the maintenance of continence. The levator ani normally relaxes under conscious control during defecation and micturition (see Figure 1–6). Tone of the levator ani muscles is extremely critical in the maintenance of continence. If the muscle tone is lax enough, the urethra is displaced and positioned so as to disrupt the balance of pressure necessary for continence.

Pressure gradients within the bladder and urethra play an important functional role in normal micturition. As the bladder initially fills, there is little rise in pressure within the bladder (intravesical pressure). When the urethral sphincter is closed, the pressure inside the urethra (intraurethral pressure) is higher than the pressure within the bladder. As long as the intraurethral pressure is higher than the

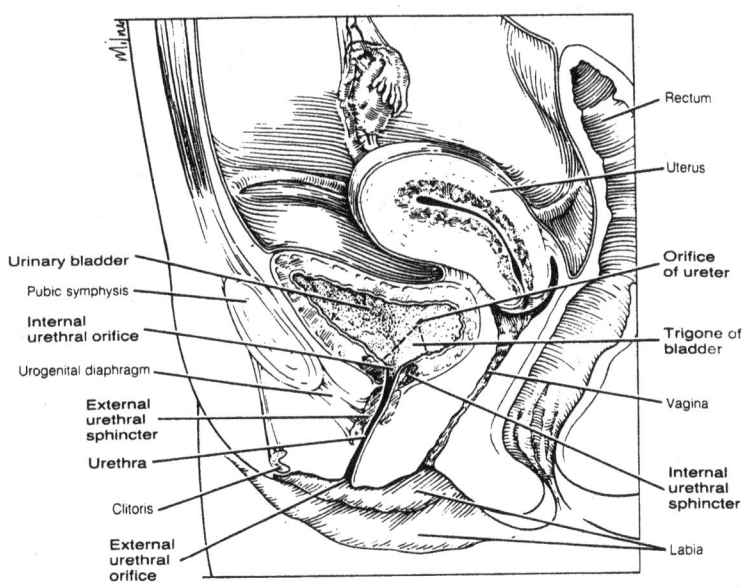

Figure 1–4 Sagittal Section of the Pelvis Showing the Female Urinary Bladder and Urethra. *Source:* Reprinted from *Basic Human Anatomy*, 3rd ed., by A. Spence, p. 582, with permission of the Benjamin/Cummings Publishing Company, © 1990.

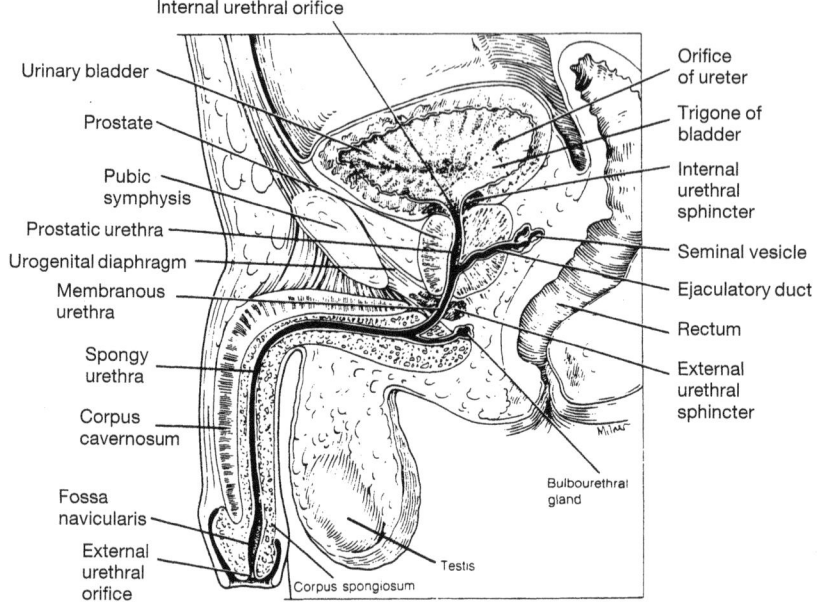

Figure 1–5 Sagittal Section of the Pelvis Showing the Male Urinary Bladder and Urethra. *Source:* Reprinted from *Basic Human Anatomy*, 3rd ed., by A. Spence, p. 582, with permission of the Benjamin/Cummings Publishing Company, © 1990.

---

intravesical pressure, continence is maintained (Claridge, 1965). During some physical activities, and with coughing, sneezing, or laughing, intra-abdominal pressure rises sharply. This rise in pressure is transmitted to both the bladder and urethra. As long as the positive pressure gradient between the bladder and urethra remains intact, no urine will leak.

SPINAL CORD

Micturition is essentially a spinal reflex that is influenced by higher centers of control in the brain (Spence, 1990). This is well illustrated by the development of continence in children. In infants, the higher center of control is not developed; therefore, when enough urine has filled the bladder to trigger the spinal reflex center, the bladder empties involuntarily. As the child's higher neurological system develops, the cortical area of the brain exerts control to inhibit emptying

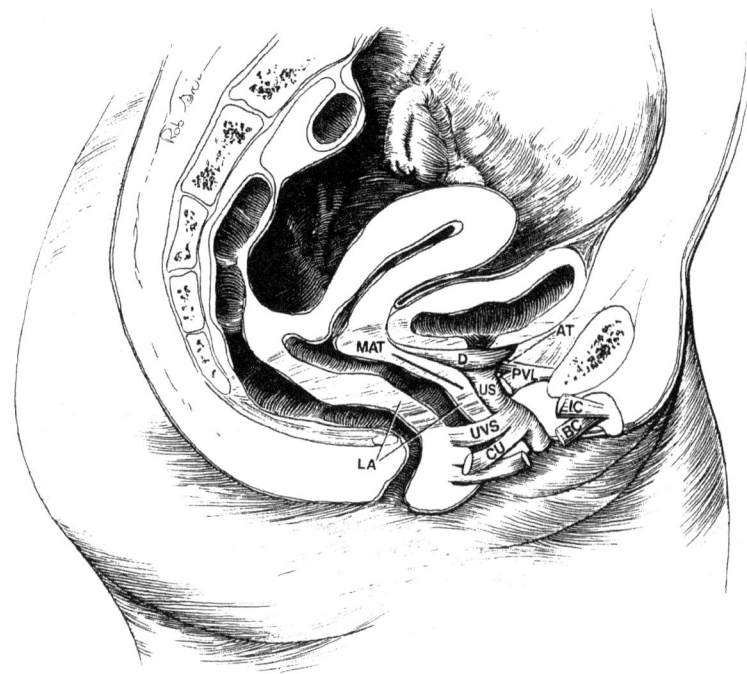

AT, arcus tendineus fasciae pelvis; BC, bulbocavernosus muscle; CU, compressor urethrae; D, detrusor loop; IC, ischiocavernosus muscle; LA, levator ani muscles; PVL, pubovesical muscle (ligaments); US, urethral sphincter; UVS, urethrovaginal sphincter

Figure 1–6 Interrelationships and Approximate Location of Paraurethral Structures. Levator ani muscles are shown as light lines running deep to the pelvic viscera. The vaginalevator attachment is shown as a darker area. *Source:* Reprinted from DeLancy, J., Correlative Study of Paraurethral Anatomy, *Obstetrics and Gynecology*, Vol. 68, No. 1, p. 299, with permission of The American College of Obstetrics and Gynecology, © 1990.

until voluntary voiding can take place. Voluntary continence is usually attained by the age of 5 years.

An intact spinal cord, therefore, is necessary for normal micturition. The spinal cord receives information from the bladder about its filling status via the afferent nerve pathways that are connected to the stretch receptors located in the bladder walls. In the normal cycle of bladder filling and emptying, the spinal cord transmits impulses to the bladder's stretch receptors along the efferent nerve pathways. These impulses keep the detrusor in a relaxed state, allowing it to continue stretching to accommodate the increasing volume of urine. Besides this linkage directly to the bladder, the spinal reflex center also transmits information to the higher center of control in the cerebral cortex. This center is called the cortical center of control.

Two areas in the spinal cord responsible for these functions are the sacral reflex center and the hypogastric plexus (see Figure 1–2). The sacral reflex center, located from S-2 to S-4, is the site of the parasympathetic activity that is responsible for bladder contraction as well as somatic nerve (pudendal nerve) innervation, which contracts and maintains the tone of the pelvic floor muscle. The hypogastric plexus, located from T-11 to L-2, receives afferent impulses from the bladder regarding fullness, and is also the site of efferent sympathetic neural activity. This activity directly relaxes the bladder and is also responsible for bladder relaxation by inhibiting parasympathetic activity (Wein, 1986). The bladder neck and urethral contraction during filling are under hypogastric plexus control as well.

When the bladder is initially filling, there is little higher level neural activity, and the person has no sensation of bladder fullness.

CORTICAL CENTER OF CONTROL

The pontine-mesencephalic gray matter, located in the brain stem, in conjunction with an area in the cerebellum (Bradley, 1986), is responsible for the coordination of the relaxation of the sphincters and contraction of the bladder to facilitate urination.

The cortical center of control is an area in the frontal lobe of the cerebral cortex responsible for the innervation of the detrusor. The primary activity of this area is to inhibit contraction of the detrusor until voluntary voiding with coordinated detrusor contraction and relaxation of sphincters takes place. After approximately 250 to 350 ml of urine has entered the bladder, the spinal reflex center alerts the cortical center via the pontine-mesencephalic gray matter. This is perceived by the person as a sensation of bladder fullness, and under normal circumstances, voluntary urination is delayed until toilet facilities are located.

CYCLE OF NORMAL MICTURITION

During the storage phase of micturition the bladder serves as a reservoir for urine. The pelvic floor muscles are contracted and the urethra is closed. The bladder passively stretches, with low intravesical pressure. The spinal reflex center monitors the activity of the detrusor expansion and relays signals to the pelvic floor to sustain or increase its tone via the somatic nerve (Palmer, 1993). As the volume of urine approaches approximately 250 to 350 ml, the intravesical pressure begins to rise sharply (see Figure 1–7). The spinal reflex center then transmits impulses to the cortical center of control. At this point, the person becomes aware of the need to void by a sensation of bladder fullness, and begins to search for a place to empty the bladder.

Once the person is prepared, the voluntary effort to void begins with the contraction of the abdomen, causing an increase in intravesical pressure. Impulses are sent from the higher centers of control to begin the second phase of micturition, bladder emptying. There is a synchronous response consisting of integrated detrusor contraction due to inhibition of sympathetic activity, elongation of the bladder neck and posterior urethra as the resistance at the bladder neck decreases and the urethral sphincter opens, and pelvic floor relaxation through inhibition of somatic nerve activity. These actions combine to cause intravesical pressure to rise, intraurethral pressure to fall, and urine to flow out of the bladder, through the urethra and out of the body. This combination of actions is micturition. Under normal conditions, there should be little urine left in the bladder after micturition. Subsequently, the detrusor resumes its relaxed storage shape, the sphincters are in the closed position, and the pelvic floor resumes its tone. At this point, the intraurethral pressure is once again higher than the intravesical pressure. This cycle of micturition is a continual process (see Figure 1–8).

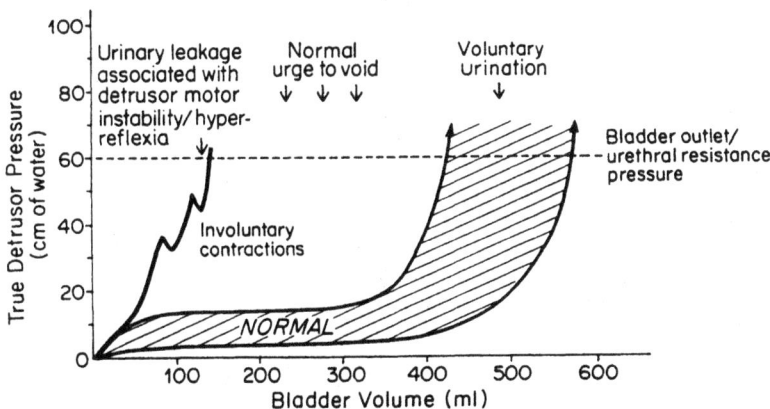

Figure 1–7 Schematic Diagram Illustrating Normal Pressure-Volume Relationships in the Bladder and the Urodynamic Phenomenon of Uninhibited or Involuntary Bladder Contractions. *Source:* Reprinted from *Essentials of Clinical Geriatrics*, 2nd ed., by R. Kane, J. Ouslander and I. Abrass, p. 144, with permission of McGraw-Hill, © 1989.

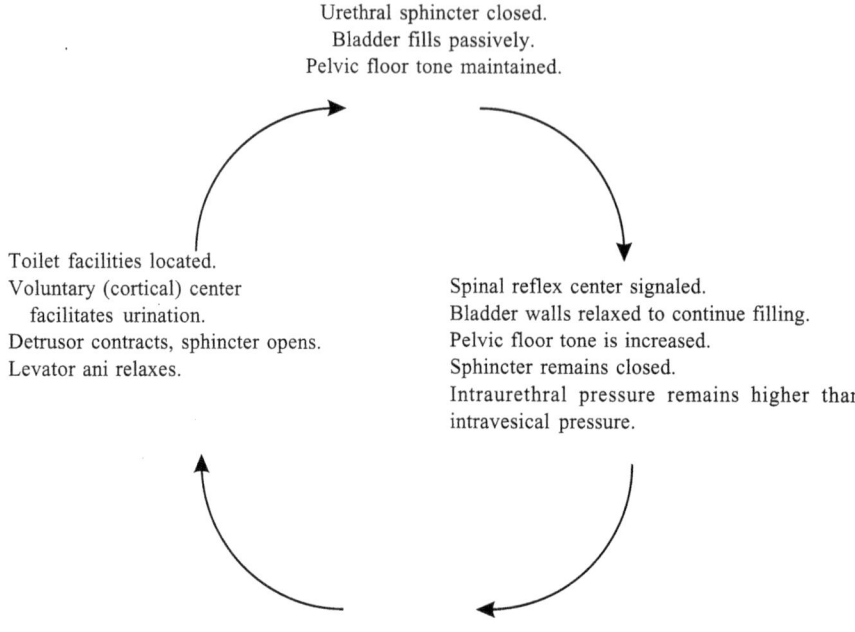

Figure 1-8 Cycle of Micturition

EFFECTS OF AGE

Normal aging changes do not cause disease, nor is urinary incontinence caused by age. Normal aging changes are gradual, and the body makes adaptations so that there is no catastrophic reaction to the alterations in function. However, although functional changes do not in themselves lead to clinical disease or disability, the older adult is more vulnerable to environmental, disease-related, or drug-induced stressors.

There are several anatomical aging changes in the renal system (see Table 1-1). The kidneys lose mass and length over the years, and by the age of 90 renal volume has decreased by 40%. There is an approximately 10% per decade decrease in renal blood flow after the age of 20. Octogenarians average a renal blood flow of approximately 300 ml/min, as compared with 600 ml/min in a young adult. Also, the proportion of body mass represented by water decreases progressively with age from 55% to 65% at age 20, to 45% to 55% at age 80. The decrease is more

Table 1-1 Common Physiological Changes

Changes	Estimated % Change at Age 80
Anatomical	
Decreased renal mass	20–30
Decreased number of functioning glomeruli	30–50
Change in characteristics of functioning glomeruli	
Functional	
Decreased renal flow	50
Increased filtration fraction	
Decreased GFR	
Decreased concentration ability	30–40
Decreased response to ADH	
Decreased ability to conserve sodium	
Increased tendency to hyperkalemia	

Note: GFR = Glomerular filtration rate; ADH = antidiuretic hormone.

Source: Reprinted from Kee, C., Age-Related Changes in the Renal System, *Geriatric Nursing*, Vol. 13, No. 2, p. 80, with permission of Mosby-Year Book, © 1992.

pronounced in women than in men because of women's lower lean body mass and higher proportion of body fat. There is also a decrease in maximal urinary concentrating ability with age. It is generally not clinically significant unless water loss is severe or the thirst mechanism is not intact.

As noted earlier, in the storage phase of the micturition cycle the bladder serves as a reservoir of urine. There is evidence that with age comes an increase of collagen in the bladder walls that may affect contractility, but what role this increase in collagen plays in micturition is not understood (Staskin, 1986).

In men, bladder neck obstruction secondary to prostatic hyperplasia is a frequent occurrence. This is due to constriction of the bladder neck and posterior urethra by prostatic enlargement. Changes in the urogenital tract in postmenopausal women are related to decreased levels of circulating estrogens. Vaginal and urethral tissues atrophy and become thinner with decreased estrogen. Also there is a decreased blood supply to the urogenital tissues, resulting in an increased possibility of urethral and vaginal irritation.

Changes in the neurological and musculoskeletal systems generally have an impact on micturition. Neurological changes include decreased reaction time and variability in the magnitude of impulses sent by the higher centers of control and the sacral reflex center, all of which may translate into a shorter time interval between the conscious awareness of the need to void and actual voiding. Muscles, especially those atrophied from disuse, have less mass and are less efficient in maintaining tone. These changes may lead to a slightly decreased bladder capacity and an increase in the number of voidings in a day, but they should not cause sudden or severe alterations in functioning. Aging does not cause incontinence. Pathological changes seen in older adults and the effects of comorbid conditions on micturition are discussed in Chapter 3.

REFERENCES

Bradley, W. (1986). Physiology of the urinary bladder. In P. Walsh, R. Gittes, A. Perlmuter, & T. Stamey (Eds.), *Campbell's urology* (5th ed.). Philadelphia: Saunders.

Brocklehurst, J. (1992). In J. Brocklehurst, R. Tallis, & H. Fillit (Eds.), *The textbook of geriatric medicine and gerontology* (4th ed.). New York: Churchill Livingstone.

Chancellor, M., & Blavais, J. (1994). Physiology of the lower urinary tract. In W. Kursh & E. McGuire (Eds.), *Female urology*. Philadelphia: Lippincott.

Claridge, M. (1965). The physiology of micturition. *British Journal of Urology, 37*, 620–623.

DeLancy, J. (1990). Anatomy and physiology of urinary continence. *Clinical Obstetrics and Gynecology, 33*, 298–307.

Guyton, A. (1991). *Basic neuroscience anatomy and physiology* (2nd ed.). Philadelphia: Saunders.

Kegel, A., & Powell, T. (1950). The physiological treatment of urinary stress incontinence. *Journal of Urology, 63*, 808–813.

Mostwin, J. (1991). Current concepts of female pelvic anatomy and physiology. *Urologic Clinics of North America, 18*, 175–195.

Palmer, M. (1993). Urinary incontinence. In V. Carrieri-Kohlman, A. Lindsey, & C. West (Eds.), *Pathophysiological phenomena in nursing* (2nd ed.). Philadelphia: Saunders.

Spence, A. (1990). *Basic human anatomy* (3rd ed.). Redwood City, CA: Benjamin/Cummings Publishing.

Staskin, D. (1986). Age-related physiologic and pathologic changes affecting lower urinary tract function. *Clinics in Geriatric Medicine, 2*, 701–710.

Wein, A. (1986). Physiology of micturition. *Clinics in Geriatric Medicine, 2*, 689–699.

CHAPTER

2

Definitions

OVERVIEW

Urinary incontinence is a term that connotes different meanings to different groups of people. To administrators of long-term care facilities, urinary incontinence is often viewed in terms of financial expenditures necessary to manage and control the odor and soiling problems. To nurses and other caregivers, urinary incontinence may be seen in terms of time spent changing clothes and bed linens rather than performing rehabilitative functions with the affected adult. The affected adult may define urinary incontinence in terms of psychological suffering and loss of control over bodily functions.

These inevitably varying perspectives on the phenomenon known as urinary incontinence tend to make efforts to address the problems of urinary continence a challenging task. Not having a common language with which to talk about the problems of urinary incontinence makes the effort to find solutions that much more difficult. For appropriate assessment and treatment of urinary incontinence to occur, there must be clear communications among clinicians, researchers, affected older adults, and caregivers. This communication cannot occur without a standard set of terminology and definitions. (See Appendix A for additional terms and conditions related to incontinence.)

Often in the past, terminology and definitions used to characterize and categorize urinary incontinence have varied considerably, both in the literature and between clinical practice settings, and often contained value-laden and subjective statements. This situation has severely hampered the sharing of clinical experience and the generalization of reports, studies, and research findings.

The lack of common terminology between health care workers and the affected patients can also cause unintentional stigmatization and shame, impeding efforts to resolve the problems associated with urinary incontinence. An early definition of incontinence was, "1. lack of restraint of the passions or appetites; free or uncontrolled indulgence of the passions or appetites; especially lack of restraint of sexual appetite, lewdness; 2. incapability of containing, holding or keeping something; 3. in medicine, the inability of any of the organs to restrain discharges of their contents, so that the discharges are involuntary; as incontinence of urine" (*Webster's New Twentieth Century Dictionary*, 1977, p. 925). However, a more recent edition of a dictionary uses a different ordering of the definitions for the word *incontinent*, i.e., "1. unable to restrain natural discharges or evacuations of urine or feces; 2. unable to contain or restrain; 3. lacking in moderation or self-control; esp. sexual desire; 4. unceasing or unrestrained" (Flexner, 1987, p. 968).

This shift in primary definition shows that the word's meanings have changed with time. However, the cohort of older adults who now may be experiencing incontinence grew up with the definition of incontinence implying immorality. Therefore, when talking with older adults, health care professionals should make clear the specific usage of the term *incontinence* when asking, "Are you incontinent?"

This chapter presents and briefly discusses current definitions used for urinary incontinence and patterns of incontinence. The International Continence Society (ICS) definitions and the definition for functional incontinence presented in this chapter are used throughout the book.

DEFINITIONS FOR URINARY INCONTINENCE

In 1992, the Agency for Health Care Policy and Research (AHCPR) published the Guideline for Urinary Incontinence in Adults to increase awareness and knowledge about this prevalent and distressing condition. This Guideline was revised in 1996. The definition provided by the AHCPR is straightforward and succinct. Urinary incontinence is defined as "involuntary loss of urine which is sufficient enough to be a problem" (Clinical Practice Guideline Panel, 1992). This definition is encompassing in scope and thus does not address the cause of incontinence or its severity. It is open to broad interpretation about what is sufficient enough to be a problem. It encompasses involuntary urine loss regardless of the environment. Voluntary or willful voiding into clothing or on furniture, walls, floors, and receptacles not designed for urinary eliminative needs is not included under this definition.

Since 1973, in an attempt to standardize terminology among researchers for the purpose of promoting generalizations and comparisons among studies, the ICS Committee on Standardisation of Terminology has developed and published terminology and definitions for types of incontinence and the methods and measurements used in the diagnosis and assessment of incontinence. This committee updates the definitions periodically, and the reader is encouraged to keep abreast of the literature for revisions in definitions and terminology. The ICS definition is similar to the AHCPR definition for incontinence. Incontinence is defined as "involuntary loss of urine which is objectively demonstrable and a social or hygienic problem" (International Continence Society [ICS] Committee on Standardisation of Terminology, 1990). Again it should be noted that severity and frequency of the involuntary loss of urine is left open to interpretation. This Committee also provided definitions for four types of incontinence in terms of a symptom—what is reported by the patient; a sign—what is objectively observed; and a condition—what is urodynamically demonstrated. The four specific types include (1) genuine stress; (2) urge, as described by the patient; (3) reflex; and (4) overflow incontinence, as evidenced by urodynamic demonstration of urine loss. Each of these four types is discussed in more detail below.

Stress Incontinence

The ICS defines stress incontinence in terms of a symptom, a sign, and a condition. The symptom is discussed as the affected person's complaint of involuntary escape of urine during any type of physical exercise. This includes changing positions, coughing, and sneezing. The sign denotes demonstrable loss of urine with physical exertion. The condition of stress incontinence is defined as an "involuntary loss of urine occurring when, in the absence of detrusor contraction, the intravesical pressure exceeds the maximum urethral pressure" (ICS Committee, 1990, p. 17). See Exhibit 2–1 for definitions.

In stress urinary incontinence, as seen in Figure 2–1, a small amount of urine escapes suddenly when the individual experiences an increase in abdominal pressure that occurs with a sneeze, a cough, or laughter. Stress incontinence often occurs in women who have given birth, although 28% of young nulliparous women athletes surveyed in one study reported episodes of incontinence during exercise (Nygaard, Thompson, Svengalis, & Albright, 1994).

The anatomical structure of a woman's short urethra and loss of urethrovesical angle as a result of a decrease in pelvic floor tone make stress incontinence more prevalent in women than in men, although men who have had a prostatectomy or perineal surgery may experience stress incontinence as well. In stress incontinence, a small amount of the urine in the bladder escapes rather than the entire contents of the bladder.

Urge Incontinence

A second type of incontinence, urge incontinence, is defined by the ICS as an "involuntary loss of urine associated with a strong desire to void (urgency)" (ICS

16   URINARY CONTINENCE

Exhibit 2-1 Definitions for Incontinence

Stress	Involuntary loss of urine, occurring when, in the absence of a detrusor contraction, the intravesical pressure exceeds the maximum urethral pressure (ICS Committee, 1990)
Urge	Involuntary loss of urine associated with a strong desire to void (urgency) (ICS Committee, 1990)
Reflex	Loss of urine due to detrusor hyper-reflexia and/or involuntary urethral relaxation in the absence of sensation usually associated with the desire to micturate (ICS Committee, 1990)
Overflow	Any involuntary loss of urine associated with overdistention of the bladder (ICS Committee, 1990)
Functional	Urinary leakage associated with inability to toilet because of impairment of cognitive and/or physical functioning, psychological unwillingness, or environmental barriers (Ouslander, 1994)

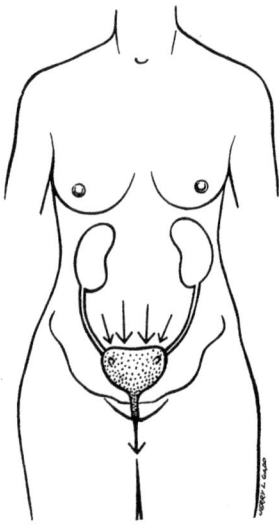

Figure 2-1 Stress Incontinence. A sudden increase in intra-abdominal pressure with a corresponding increase in intravesical pressure exceeding intraurethral pressure forces urine out.

Committee, 1990, p. 17). The urgency described by the patient may be associated with sensory urgency (hypersensitivity) or it may be associated with the overactive function of the detrusor, also referred to as motor urgency (see Figures 2–2 and 2–3).

An example of sensory urgency is the strong desire to void associated with intense emotional excitation or nervousness. An example of motor urgency is when a person has uninhibited detrusor contractions of sufficient magnitude to cause urine to empty from the bladder.

A person with urge incontinence is aware of the need to void, but is unable to prevent the bladder from emptying its contents until toilet facilities are reached. Two related terms defined by the ICS are *unstable detrusor* and *detrusor hyperreflexia*. An unstable detrusor "is one that is shown objectively to contract, spontaneously or on provocation, during the filling phase while the patient is attempting to inhibit micturition" (ICS Committee, 1990, p. 16). Detrusor hyperreflexia is defined as "overactivity due to disturbance of the nervous control mechanisms" (ICS Committee, 1990, p. 16). This term is to be used when there is a relevant neurological disorder.

One term related to urge incontinence found in older literature was *unstable bladder*, which had been used to describe motor urge incontinence. Another term previously used was *uninhibited neurogenic bladder*. This term was formerly used to describe incontinence resulting from a lesion in the cerebral cortex in which sensation of bladder fullness was intact but inhibitory control was absent. Incontinence was characterized by the sensation of the need to void followed almost immediately by the uncontrolled contraction of the detrusor.

Reflex Incontinence

Reflex incontinence is defined by the ICS as "the loss of urine due to hyperreflexia and/or involuntary urethral relaxation in the absence of sensation usually associated with the desire to micturate" (ICS Committee, 1990, p. 17).

Reflex incontinence, or *unconscious incontinence,* occurs in paraplegics; there is no sensory awareness of the need to void. Constant postmicturition dribbling without an overt neurologic dysfunction also is considered unconscious incontinence (Fantl, Newman, & Colling et al., 1996).

The terms *spastic bladder, upper motor neuron,* and *central neurogenic bladder* were used in the literature to describe the incontinence that occurs when the brain no longer receives signals from the spinal cord. The resultant bladder reflex causes an overactive and poorly coordinated detrusor contraction. Rather than being large and flaccid, the bladder is small and unable to hold large amounts

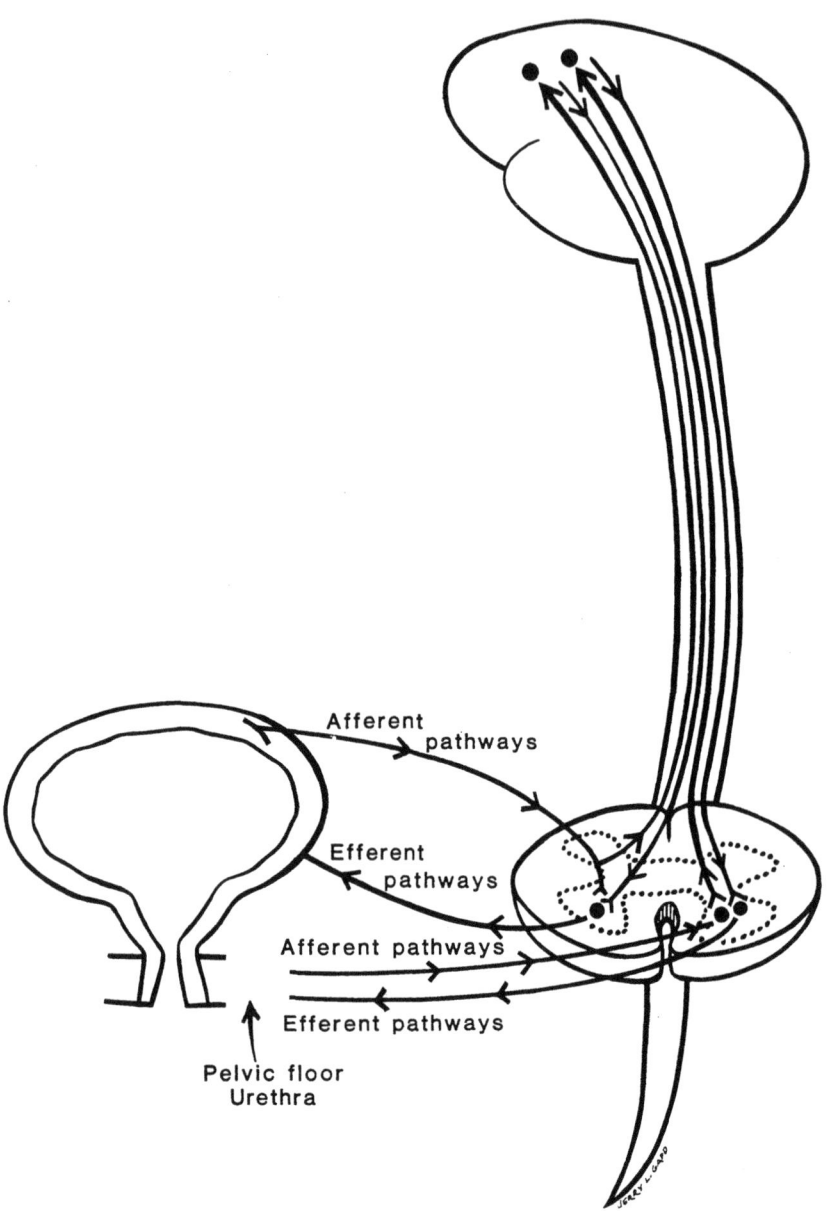

Figure 2–2 Sensory Urge Incontinence. Sensation to void is present with no uninhibited detrusor contractions.

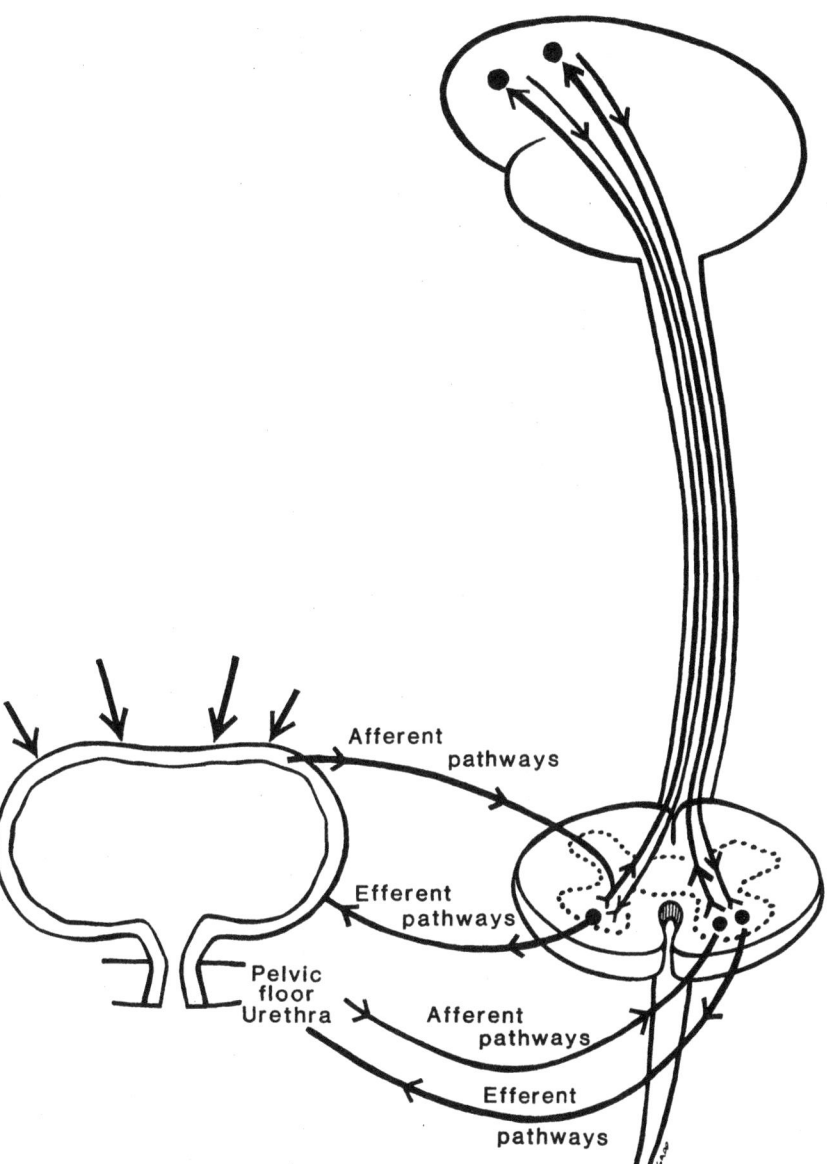

Figure 2-3 Motor Urge Incontinence. Sensation to void is present, but the individual is unable to inhibit detrusor contraction.

of urine. The individual is unaware of the need to void, and urine escapes without conscious knowledge (see Figure 2–4). The term *reflex incontinence* will not be used throughout the text.

Overflow Incontinence

The final type of incontinence defined by the ICS is overflow incontinence. It is defined as "any involuntary loss of urine associated with overdistention of the bladder" (ICS Committee, 1990, p. 17). Because of the overdistention, the pressure within the bladder, the intravesical pressure, is greater than the pressure in the urethra. As described in Chapter 1, continence is maintained when the urethral pressure stays higher than the pressure in the bladder. In overflow incontinence, even when the bladder is filled to capacity, the detrusor does not contract. As a result, urine dribbles out because of the continuing rise in the pressure in the bladder, which eventually becomes greater than the pressure in the urethra (see Figure 2–5). The bladder can overdistend and urine can overflow for several reasons. A disruption at the bladder outlet as in prostatic obstruction or fecal impaction can prevent urine from emptying. Also, the afferent pathways that normally carry impulses of bladder fullness to the spinal cord may no longer do so because of disease or injury. Because of the outlet obstruction or disruption in nerve transmission, the bladder appears flaccid and distended with urine, which finally results in overflow incontinence.

The terms *atonic bladder* and *lower motor neuron bladder* were previously used to describe overflow incontinence resulting from a disruption affecting the sacral reflex center.

Functional Incontinence

One final type of incontinence—functional incontinence—is not defined by the ICS, although it has been defined in the literature. Williams and Pannill (1982) noted that people who normally can control micturition become incontinent due to factors outside the urinary tract, such as mobility impairment. Ouslander (1994) defined functional incontinence as "urinary leakage associated with inability to toilet because of impairment of cognitive and/or physical functioning, psychological unwillingness or environmental barriers" (p. 151).

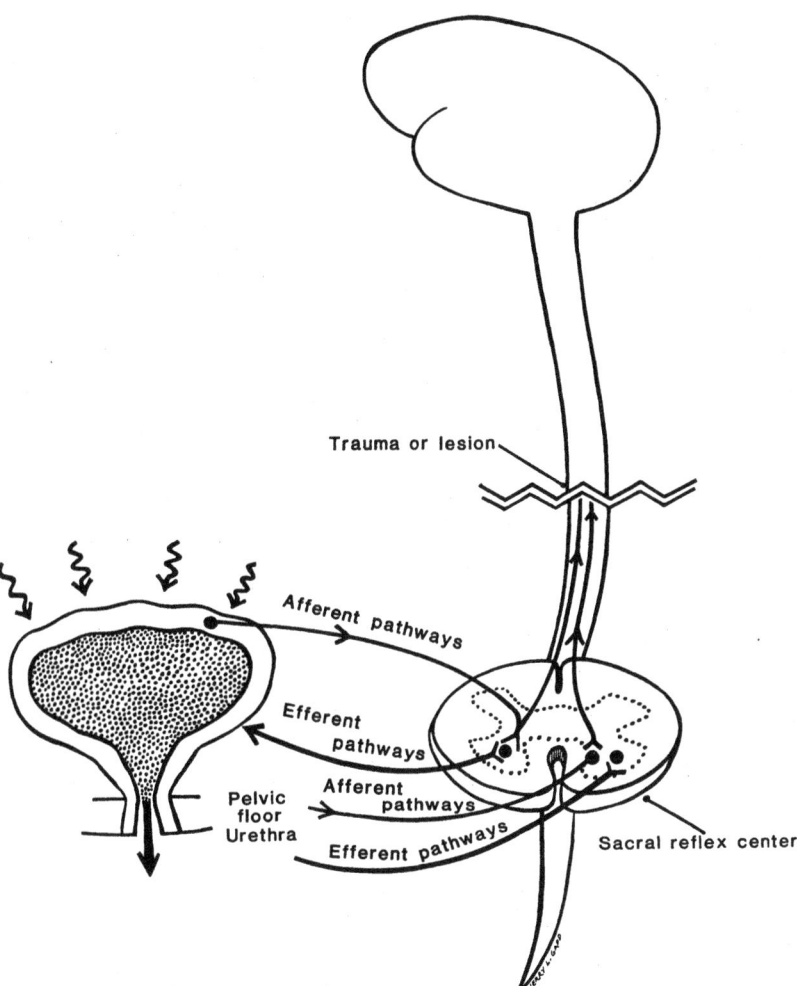

Figure 2–4 Reflex Incontinence. No sensation to void is present. Detrusor contraction is controlled by the sacral reflex center.

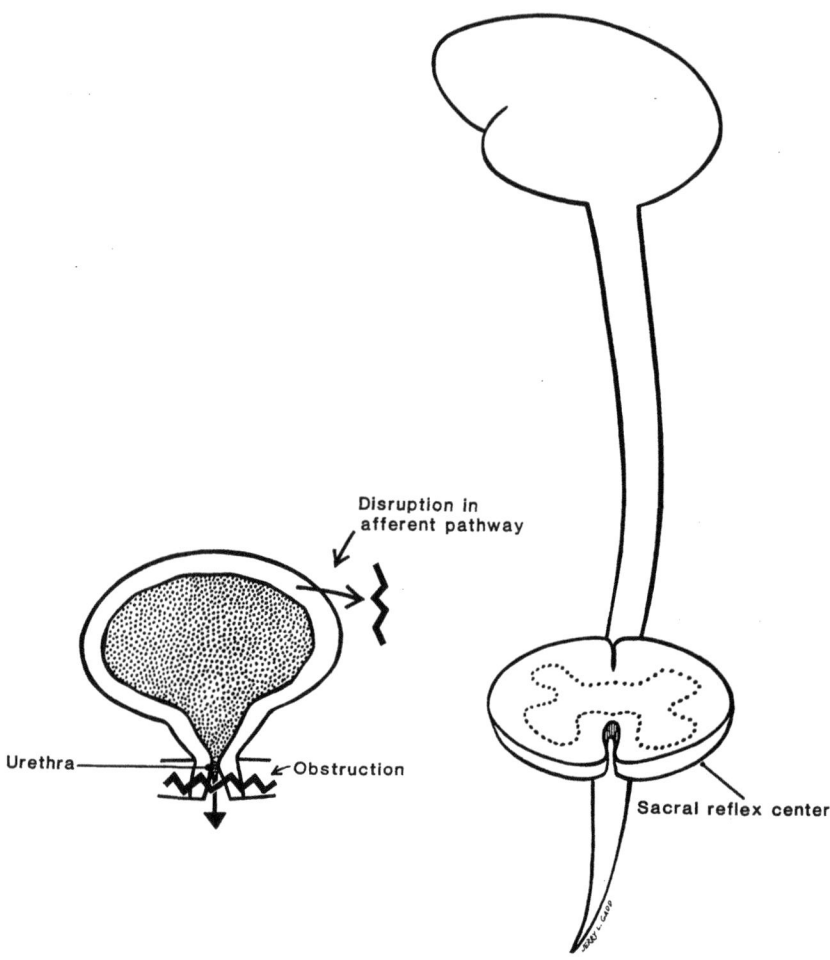

Figure 2-5 Overflow Incontinence. If the disruption is in the afferent pathway to the sacral reflex center, no sensation to void is present, and the bladder overflows. Alternatively, an obstruction at the outlet can cause bladder distention and overflow incontinence.

PATTERNS OF INCONTINENCE

Besides types of incontinence, patterns of incontinence have been defined as well. For some people, urinary incontinence may be a longstanding problem. In a survey of over 10,000 older adults, the average length of time for being incontinent was 9 years (Jeter & Wagner, 1990). Incontinence that has persisted is called established incontinence.

In contrast, transient incontinence (also referred to as acute incontinence) appears suddenly, often accompanying a change in health, medication regimen, or environment. The terms *established* and *transient* are used throughout the text when patterns of incontinence are discussed. Chapter 3 provides a full discussion of the causes of established and transient incontinence.

REFERENCES

Clinical Practice Guideline Panel. (1992). *Clinical practice guideline: Urinary incontinence in adults* (AHCPR Pub. No. 92-0038). Rockville, MD: Agency for Health Care Policy and Research, Public Health Service, U.S. Department of Health and Human Services.

Fantl, J.A., Newman, D.K., & Colling, J. et al. (1996). *Urinary incontinence in adults: Acute and chronic management. Clinical practice guideline no. 2, 1996 update.* (AHCPR Pub. No. 96-0682). Rockville, MD: Agency for Health Care Policy and Research, Public Health Service, U.S. Department of Health and Human Services.

Flexner, S. (Ed.). (1987). *Random House dictionary of the English language* (2nd ed.). New York: Random House.

International Continence Society Committee on Standardisation of Terminology. (1990). The standardisation of terminology of the lower urinary tract function. *British Journal of Obstetrics and Gynaecology, 97* (Suppl. 6).

Jeter, K., & Wagner, D. (1990). Incontinence in the American home: A survey of 36,500 people. *Journal of the American Geriatrics Society, 38*, 379–383.

Nygaard, I., Thompson, F., Svengalis, S., & Albright, J. (1994). Urinary incontinence in elite nulliparous athletes. *Obstetrics and Gynecology, 84*, 183–187.

Ouslander, J. (1994). Incontinence. In R. Kane, J. Ouslander, & I. Abrass (Eds.). *Essentials of clinical geriatrics* (3rd ed.). New York: McGraw-Hill.

Webster's new twentieth century dictionary. (1977). New York: Collins World.

Williams, M., & Pannill, F. (1982). Urinary incontinence in the elderly. *Annals of Internal Medicine, 97*, 895–907.

CHAPTER

3

Associated Factors and Causes

Urinary incontinence is a complex phenomenon involving disruptions in the filling, storage, and/or emptying of urine. There are multiple causes and factors associated with incontinence; however, age alone does not cause incontinence (see Exhibit 3–1). Understanding the underlying pathophysiology of incontinence is an important prerequisite to the assessment, classification, and treatment of incontinence.

Besides discussing the causes and associated factors of incontinence, this chapter briefly reviews the prevalence of incontinence in various health care settings. In this chapter the causes and the factors associated with the different types of established incontinence have been classified into three broad categories: urogenital, neurological, and environmental. Although presented separately, there may be more than one cause or associated factor and more than one type of incontinence present.

PREVALENCE OF INCONTINENCE

The involuntary loss of urine is a common problem. More than 13 million adult Americans report experiencing involuntary urine loss (Fantl, Newman, & Colling et al., 1996). Even nulliparous physically fit young women have reported the symptom of incontinence. Nygaard, Thompson, Svengalis, and Albright (1994) stated that women with the average age of 20 years reported to have experienced incontinence with vigorous exercise. Differentiating between the symptom of incontinence, an episodic event, and the condition of incontinence, an ongoing problem, is important to the clinician and is discussed in more detail in Chapter 4.

The prevalence of incontinence varies by health care setting and gender (see Table 3–1).

Exhibit 3–1 Causes of Urinary Incontinence

Type	Cause
Stress	• Incompetent urethra • Weak pelvic floor musculature
Urge	Lower Urinary Tract: • Urinary tract infection • Cystitis • Bladder tumor • Bladder stones Neurological: • Cerebrovascular accident • Dementia • Parkinson's disease • Normal pressure hydrocephalus • Multiple sclerosis • Spinal cord tumor/lesion
Overflow	Outlet Obstruction: • Prostatic hyperplasia • Fecal impaction Chronic Myogenic Decompensation: • Peripheral neuropathy
Functional	• Impaired mobility • Severe dementia • Communication difficulties • Depression • Hostility • Caregiver, toilet, and/or toilet substitutes unavailable

Source: Adapted from Palmer, M., Urinary Incontinence, in *Pathophysiological Phenomena in Nursing: Human Response to Illness* by V. Carrieri-Kohlman, A. Lindsay and C. West, eds., p. 225, with permission of W.B. Saunders, © 1993.

Long-Term Care Setting

Residents of long-term care facilities have the highest reported prevalence; approximately 50% of residents are incontinent of urine (Fantl et al., 1996). Impairment of mobility and cognition have long been reported as factors associated with incontinence (Resnick & Yalla, 1987a; Yu et al., 1990). Palmer, German, and Ouslander (1991) identified risk factors for incontinence in the long-term care setting after the first year of admission to be dementia, mobility impairment, male

Table 3–1 Prevalence of Urinary Incontinence

Study	Population Sample	Definition of Incontinence	Prevalence
Setting: Acute Care			
Sullivan & Lindsay (1984)	N = 315 (pts 65+ yr) admitted over a 6-wk period	Any inappropriate loss of urine, regardless of amount or frequency Included use of external catheter; excluded indwelling catheter	19%
Sier, Ouslander, & Orzeck (1987)	N = 363 (pts 65+ yr) admitted over a 14-wk period	One or more episodes of incontinence documented on Incontinence Monitoring Record while hospitalized	Age: 65–74 = 24% 75+ = 48%
Massachusetts Medical Society (1991)	N = 41.4 million hospital discharge records (Medicare A)	First mention of incontinence in discharge records	Women: 16.6 Men: 10.1 (per 10,000 population)
Setting: Long-Term Care			
Ouslander, Kane, & Abrass (1982)	N = 842 (pts 65+ yr) from seven nursing homes	Any uncontrolled leakage of urine, regardless of amount or frequency	50%
Ouslander & Fowler (1985)	N = 7,853, all VA patients in 90 nursing home facilities	Any uncontrolled leakage of urine, regardless of amount or frequency	41%
Hing and Sekscenski (1986)	N = 1.4 million (pts 55+ yr)	Difficulty controlling bladder	10.7% bladder only; 32.5% bladder and bowel
Palmer, German, & Ouslander (1991)	N = 430 (pt 60+ yr) newly admitted nursing home residents	Incontinent during the day	39% at 2 wk after admission; 41% 1 yr after admission

continues

Table 3-1 continued

Study	Population Sample	Definition of Incontinence	Prevalence
Setting: Community			
Diokno, Brock, Brown, & Herzog (1986)	N = 1,955 (adults 60+ yr)	Any uncontrolled urine loss in the prior 12 mo without regard to severity	30% average (18.9% males, 37.7% females)
Harris (1986)	N = 5,637 (adults 65+ yr) who answered questions regarding urinary problems on the National Health Interview Survey	Includes those with any difficulty controlling urination as well as those with catheters	9%
Mohide, Pringle, Robertson, & Chambers (1988)	N = 2,801 (avg age 74 yr) patients of four home care programs	Involuntary urine loss in association with strong desire to void, physical exertion; no apparent sensation of need to void if irregular toileting occurred	22%
Wetle et al. (1995)	N = 3,809 (study participants 65+ yr)	"Difficulty holding urine until they can get to a toilet"	28%

Source: Adapted from Palmer, M., Urinary Incontinence, in *Pathophysiological Phenomena in Nursing: Human Response to Illness* by V. Carrieri-Kohlman, A. Lindsay and C. West, eds., p. 223, with permission of W.B. Saunders, © 1993.

---

gender, and behavioral problems in adjusting to the institution. Although the prevalence of incontinence was higher in women in this and many other studies, previously continent men developed incontinence at a higher rate than did previously continent women. The reason or reasons why men developed incontinence at a higher rate is not clear. It may be that men are in poorer health upon admission to long-term care facilities than are women. More research is needed to understand fully how and why incontinence develops.

Home Care Setting

The profiles of individuals in the home care setting are similar to those of residents in long-term care facilities. As noted in Table 3–1, Mohide et al. (1988) found a 22% prevalence of incontinence among 2,801 patients receiving services from home care agencies. The most frequent concomitant conditions in this population were cerebrovascular disease, arthritis, and heart disease. These individuals also had functional impairments, especially related to mobility.

Community Setting

Community-dwelling elderly have a lower prevalence of incontinence; usually 15% to 35% are the reported ranges (Fantl et al., 1996). Incontinence in this population has been associated with poor health (Herzog, Fultz, Brock, Brown, & Diokno, 1988). Wetle and her colleagues (1995) noted that the presence of depression, a chronic cough, fecal incontinence, and difficulties in activities of daily living were some of the factors associated with difficulty in holding urine. Tinetti, Inouye, Gill, and Doucette (1995) found hearing and vision impairment, anxiety, and upper and lower extremity impairment as predisposing factors for falling and urinary incontinence. These authors noted that impairments in several domains—physical, psychological, and sensory—indicate a complex mechanism in the development of incontinence and functional dependence.

Acute Care Setting

In the acute care setting, incontinence can go undetected by the nursing staff. Palmer, Bone, Fahey, Mamon, and Steinwachs (1992) found that nurses did not identify younger (between the ages of 60 and 64 years) and independent incontinent patients, while they more frequently identified the functionally impaired and men of advanced years.

Understanding that incontinence can appear alternatively as a sign, symptom, and/or condition is important when one assesses the underlying causes of incontinence. Knowledge of the magnitude of the problem and the risk factors for incontinence in different populations can help in the assessment and treatment of incontinence, in providing staff training and development of treatment protocols, and in anticipating the types of resources needed for treatment and care.

PATHOPHYSIOLOGY OF INCONTINENCE

Sufficient disruptions or defects in either the function or the structures of the components responsible for micturition can cause urinary incontinence. Depending on the type and location of the pathophysiology, these disruptions may occur in the storage/filling or emptying phases of micturition (see Figure 3–1). When there are combined or mixed types of incontinence present, disruptions can occur in both the storage and emptying phase of micturition. For example, a woman with a lax pelvic floor that causes sphincter incompetence experiences a disruption in the storage phase of micturition. However, if she also has peripheral neuropathy secondary to diabetes mellitus, she may also experience decreased contractility of the detrusor, causing a disruption in the emptying phase of micturition.

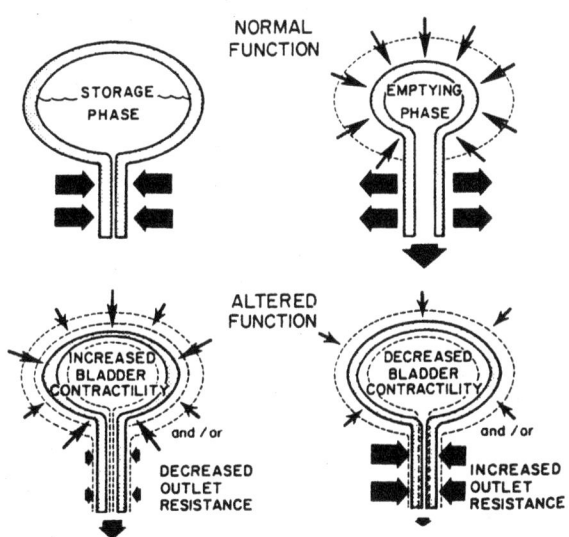

Figure 3–1 Pathophysiology of Urinary Incontinence. *Source:* Reprinted from Wyman, J., Incontinence and Related Problems, in *Clinical Gerontological Nursing: A Guide to Advanced Practice* by W. Chenitz, J. Stone and S. Salisbury, eds., p. 184, with permission of W.B. Saunders, © 1991.

CAUSES OF TRANSIENT INCONTINENCE

Transient incontinence is a pattern of incontinence that appears suddenly in an otherwise continent person. The causes of the incontinence are potentially treatable. Two acronyms, DRIP and DIAPPERS, have been developed to aid in the identification of transient incontinence (Exhibits 3–2 and 3–3).

Transient incontinence can be triggered by acute urinary tract infections, temporary confusion or delirium, immobilization, sudden or worsening illness, and medications. Once the underlying disorder is reversed or treated, the incontinence usually disappears. If left untreated, transient incontinence may evolve into established incontinence. Assessment of transient incontinence is discussed in Chapter 4.

Exhibit 3–2 Causes of Acute and Reversible Forms of Incontinence

D	Delirium
R	Restricted mobility, retention
I	Infection,* Inflammation,* Impaction (fecal)
P	Polyuria,† pharmaceuticals

*Acute symptomatic urinary tract infection, atrophic vaginitis, or urethritis.
†Hyperglycemia, volume-expanded states causing excessive nocturia (e.g., congestive heart failure, venous insufficiency).

Source: Reprinted from *Essentials of Clinical Geriatrics*, 3rd ed., by R. Kane, J. Ouslander and I. Abrass, p. 154, with permission of McGraw-Hill, © 1994.

Exhibit 3–3 Causes of Transient Incontinence

D	elirium/confusional state
I	nfection-urinary (symptomatic)
A	trophic urethritis/vaginitis
P	harmaceuticals
P	sychologic, especially depression
E	xcessive urine output (e.g., congestive heart failure, hyperglycemia)
R	estricted mobility
S	tool impaction

Source: Reprinted from Resnick, N., and Yalla, S., Evaluation and Management of Urinary Incontinence, in *Campbell's Urology*, 6th ed., by P. Walsh, A. Retisk, T. Stamey and E. Vaughn, eds., p. 644, with permission of W.B. Saunders, © 1992.

UROGENITAL CAUSES AND FACTORS

Prostatic Enlargement: Men

One of the most common urologic causes of incontinence in men is prostatic enlargement. The prostate gland is situated below the bladder and encircles the urethra (see Figure 3–2). A major constituent of seminal fluid is produced in the prostate gland. As men age, the prostate gland enlarges. More than 50% of 60-year-old men and more than 90% of 85-year-old men have microscopic evidence of benign prostatic hyperplasia. Of these, approximately half will have enlargement of the prostate gland (Clinical Practice Guideline Panel, 1994). It is estimated that half of these men develop macroscopic enlargement of the prostate gland and experience urinary symptoms. These symptoms can be grouped as obstructive symptoms and irritative symptoms (Wein, 1993) (see Exhibit 3–4).

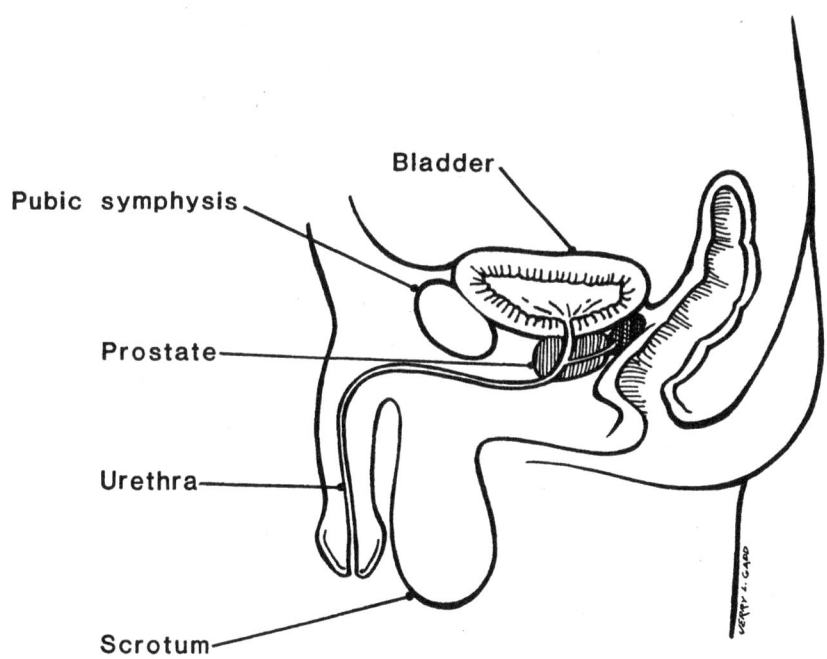

Figure 3–2 Lateral View of the Male Genitourinary System

Exhibit 3-4 Urinary Symptoms in Men with Benign Prostatic Hyperplasia

Obstructive Symptoms (Emptying Phase)	Irritative Symptoms (Storage/Filling Phase)
• Hesitancy • Decreased stream • Feeling of incomplete voiding • Postvoiding dribble • Urinary retention	• Increased daytime frequency • Nocturia • Urgency • Incontinence associated with involuntary bladder contractions

Source: Compiled from Wein, A., Criteria for Assessing Outcome Following Intervention for Benign Prostatic Hypertrophy, in *Prostate Disease* by H. Lepor and R. Lawson, eds., W.B. Saunders, © 1993.

The enlarged prostate can cause obstruction at the bladder neck, resulting in a sensation of incomplete emptying. In response to an obstruction, the detrusor thickens (hypertrophies) and there may be more forceful and uninhibited contractions of the detrusor, leading to urgency (Wein, 1993). Some men experience severe or complete obstruction of the bladder neck whereby the bladder cannot be emptied of urine, resulting in overflow incontinence. This may also occur in conjunction with the use of a medication with anticholinergic effects, which increases urethral resistance (Zawada, 1985).

Stress, urge, and total incontinence may occur after surgical treatment for benign prostatic hyperplasia (Clinical Practice Guideline Panel, 1994). The prevalence of this complication is infrequent (Appell, 1994). After transurethral resection of the prostate (TURP), the most common surgical treatment for benign prostatic hyperplasia, 2.1% of men experience stress incontinence, 1.9% of men experience urge incontinence, and 1.0% of men experience total incontinence.

Several factors may contribute to the occurrence of incontinence after surgical treatment of benign prostatic hyperplasia. Surgical trauma to the distal urethral mechanism can lead to sphincter incompetency (Raz, 1978), disrupting the filling and storing phase of micturition, resulting in stress incontinence. Also, prior to surgery, the detrusor exerts uninhibited, forceful contractions in an attempt to overcome the obstruction at the bladder neck and to empty the bladder (Barry, 1993). These powerful contractions, although no longer necessary postoperatively, may continue for some time after the surgery, causing transient urge incontinence.

Pelvic Prolapse: Women

The normal positions of the female urogenital structures are displayed in Figure 3-3. The bladder is adjacent to the anterior vaginal wall and is above the

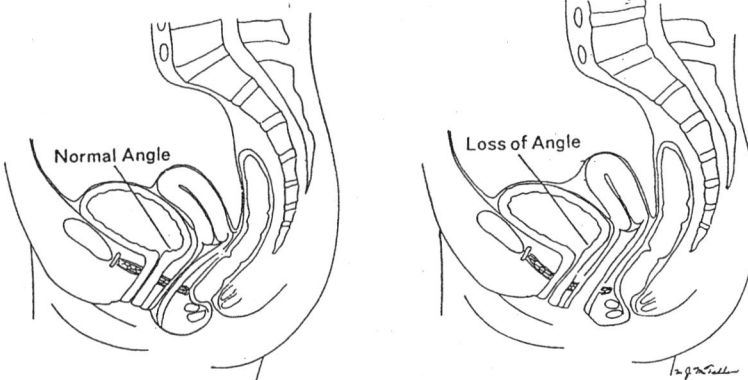

Figure 3-3 Anatomical Changes in Women Due to Birth Trauma That Contribute to Stress Incontinence. *Source:* Reprinted from Zawada, E., Voiding Problems in the Elderly: Functional Disorders of the Lower Urinary Tract, in *Geriatric Nephrology and Urology* by E. Zawada and D. Sica, eds., p. 318, with permission of Mosby-Year Book, © 1985.

urethrovesical junction. The posterior angle formed at the junction of the bladder and urethra normally measures between 90 and 100 degrees. This angle, also known as the posterior urethrovesical angle, is crucial to continence (Shortlife & Stamey, 1986). This angle can be reduced due to trauma from birth, anterior vaginal surgery, and prolapse of other urogenital structures, resulting in incontinence. Vaginal delivery is the most common reason for prolapse of urogenital organs and incontinence (Wall, Norton, & DeLancey, 1993).

Prolapses of the bladder (cystocele), urethra (urethrocele), bladder and urethra (cystourethrocele), rectum (rectocele), and the peritoneal sac that lies behind the uterus and in front of the rectum (enterocele) may contribute to incontinence. Prolapse of these organs can cause poor pelvic support of the bladder and urethra, resulting in their lying below their normal positions, leading to defects in the transmission of pressures. Stress incontinence is often a result of a cystocele. Other associated urinary symptoms may occur as well (e.g., frequency, urgency, or obstruction of bladder emptying). The structural defect of a cystocele lies in the anterior vaginal wall, not in the bladder (Wall et al., 1993), and should be described as an anterior vaginal wall prolapse (Bump et al., 1995).

Pelvic Floor Musculature: Women

When the muscles of the pelvic floor are weak or lax in the absence of a prolapse, the proximal urethra, the portion of the urethra closest to the bladder, lies below the pelvic floor. Consequently, the urethral pressure does not rise in correspondence with the rise in the bladder pressure. Urine empties from the bladder, the area of higher pressure, to the urethra, the area of lower pressure.

The underlying pathophysiology of stress incontinence in some women may be due to defects in urogenital structures, damage to neural pathways, and tearing of connective tissue that result in changes in pressure gradients (Wall et al., 1993). Ulmsten (1995) noted that there are two major defects in stress incontinence: weak or damaged pubourethral ligaments (pelvic floor) or a defective vaginal wall, or a combination of both.

Hormonal Influences: Women

The dramatic reduction of circulating estrogens in postmenopausal women may play a role in the development of incontinence (Fantl, Cardozo, McClish, et al., 1994). The urethra, bladder neck, and muscles in the pelvic floor have hormone receptors, as does the vagina (Ulmsten, 1995). Lack of estrogen is linked to a reduction in the collagen content in the surrounding connective tissue (Rekers, Drogendijk, Valkenburg, & Riphagen, 1992). When replacement estrogen is given, there is an improvement of the urethral closure mechanism and restoration of vaginal flora and pH, reducing risks for urinary tract infections (Versi, 1990). When atrophy of urogenital tissue occurs due to the decreased level of estrogen, symptoms of urethritis and vaginitis often appear. Besides incontinence, other urogenital symptoms may appear after menopause, including urgency, frequency, and dysuria (Rekers et al., 1992).

Other Urogenital Causes of Incontinence

Resnick and Yalla (1987b) first identified a type of detrusor abnormality in nursing home residents, detrusor hyperactivity with impaired contractility (DHIC). Individuals with DHIC experience frequent but ineffective involuntary detrusor contractions. There is poor emptying of urine, resulting in high residual urine volumes in the bladder. These individuals may be at risk for developing urinary retention, especially if a concomitant condition is present, such as fecal impaction or use of anticholinergic medications. In women, DHIC may be misdiagnosed as stress incontinence if an uninhibited contraction is initiated by a stress-provocative maneuver. In men, DHIC may be misdiagnosed as prostatism because the two conditions share the same symptoms: urgency, large residual volumes, and weak flow rate (Resnick & Yalla, 1992). The etiology of this disorder is not clear.

Resnick and Yalla (1987b) suggested that there may be impaired detrusor neuromuscular transmissions or myopathic processes occurring.

Acute urinary tract infections can contribute to transient incontinence. The inflammation from the infection causes irritation to the bladder wall. This in turn causes signals from the bladder wall receptors to be sent to the sacral reflex center. Thus, the neurological component of the cycle of micturition is accelerated, creating the sensation of urgency. Chronic bacteriuria, the presence of bacteria in the urine, is common in older adults. However, researchers have not established a relationship between the presence of chronic asymptomatic bacteriuria and urinary incontinence (Fantl et al., 1996).

NEUROLOGICAL CAUSES

The structures necessary for micturition and their innervation are displayed in Figure 3–4.

The bladder has stretch receptors, sensitive to the filling of urine, located within its muscular wall. As the bladder fills, impulses are sent along the afferent autonomic nerve pathway, the bladder sensory nerve, to the spinal reflex arc (see Figure 3–5).

A signal is returned along the efferent pathway, the detrusor motor fiber, to inhibit muscular contraction of the detrusor and to continue stretching of the detrusor to accommodate more urine. Sensory signals relaying information about bladder filling are also sent from the sacral reflex center to the brain stem and cerebral cortex (see Figure 3–5). After approximately 250 to 350 ml of urine has accumulated in the bladder, the person is aware of the need to void and conscious inhibition of emptying is necessary.

Several areas in the brain are responsible for the voluntary, or conscious, control of micturition. The purpose of conscious control is twofold: to postpone emptying of the bladder until socially appropriate, and to provide a mechanism of smooth, efficient emptying through synchronization of detrusor contraction and urethral relaxation. An interference or lesion at any point of the neurological control of micturition can cause incontinence. It should be noted that specific areas and nerve pathways that control bladder function have not been clearly identified by researchers.

There are several neurological causes of incontinence, including suprasacral lesions, sacral spinal lesions, and increased afferent loop stimulation (see Exhibit 3–5). It should be noted, however, that certain conditions may cause more than one type of incontinence. As an example, a person with a fecal impaction may have a bladder outlet obstruction that results in ineffective emptying but also may

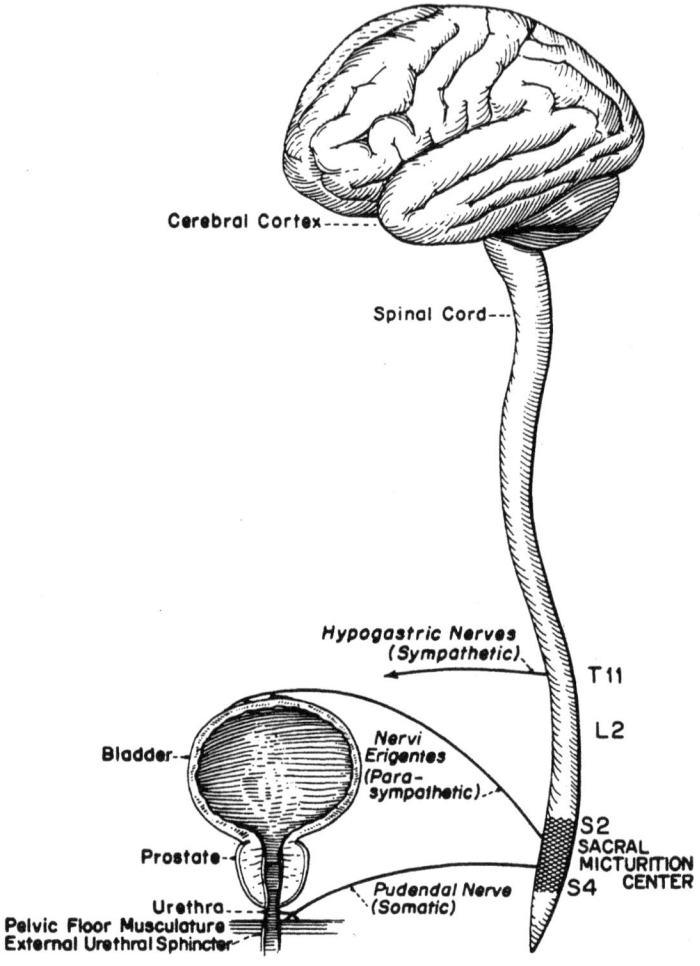

Figure 3–4 Structural Components of Normal Micturition. *Source:* Reprinted from *Essentials of Clinical Geriatrics*, 3rd ed., by R. Kane, J. Ouslander and I. Abrass, p. 142, with permission of McGraw-Hill, © 1994.

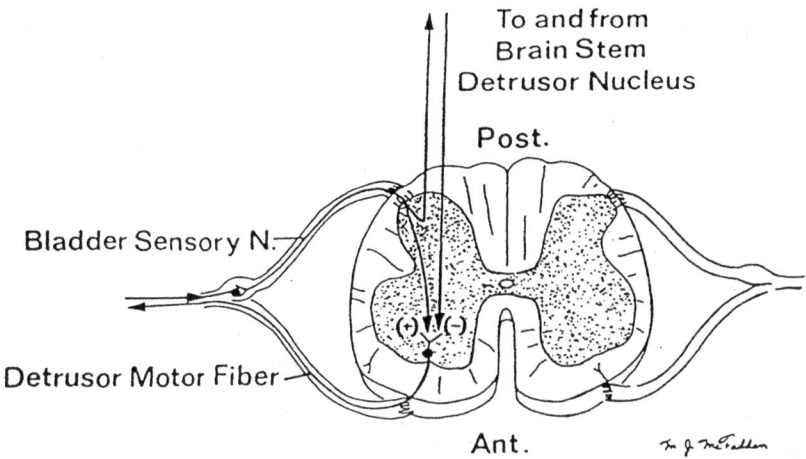

Figure 3–5 Neural Pathways Mediating Increased Afferent Loop Stimulation to the Detrusor Motor Fibers. *Source:* Reprinted from Zawada, E., Voiding Problems in the Elderly: Functional Disorders of the Lower Urinary Tract, in *Geriatric Nephrology and Urology* by E. Zawada and D. Sica, p. 322, with permission of Mosby-Year Book, © 1985.

---

have increased afferent loop stimulation due to the pressure placed on the bladder by the distended bowel.

Suprasacral Spinal Lesions

Suprasacral spinal lesions usually lead to detrusor hyper-reflexia due to disruptions in the inhibition of micturition. Suprasacral spinal lesions occur in the cerebral cortex, subcortex, and suprasacral spinal cord (Resnick & Yalla, 1992). Urinary incontinence occurring after a cerebrovascular accident (CVA) can be due to cerebral lesions that affect structures and nerve pathways responsible for micturition (urge incontinence) and to loss of mobility (functional incontinence) (Motola & Badlani, 1990). Brain injury due to surgery or trauma (e.g., falls) can also cause incontinence, depending on the severity and location of the damage. A lesion or damage in the frontal area of the cerebral cortex responsible for voluntary control could cause urge incontinence. For example, ascending sensory signals from the sacral reflex center arrive at the proper destination in the cortex, but the

Exhibit 3–5 Neurological Causes of Incontinence

Cause	Mechanism	Disruption
Suprasacral spinal lesions • Cerebrovascular accident • Brain injuries, tumors • Parkinson's disease • Alzheimer's disease • Multiple sclerosis • Suprasacral spinal transections • Normal pressure hydrocephalus • Neoplasms	Defects in inhibitory control, leading to detrusor hyperreflexia and *urge incontinence*	Storage phase
Sacral spinal cord lesions • Diabetes mellitus • Tabes dorsalis • Alcoholic neuropathy • Sacral spinal cord lesions • Disk compression • Pernicious anemia	Impaired sensory limb of reflex arc or lesions along afferent tracks to the brain, leading to detrusor inadequacy and *overflow incontinence*	Emptying phase
Increased afferent loop stimulation • Urinary tract infection • Uterine prolapse • Prostatic hyperplasia • Fecal impaction • Neoplasm	Increased bladder sensory activity transmitted to spinal detrusor motor fiber exceeds inhibitory control of cortex, leading to *urge incontinence*	Storage phase

inhibitory response is not sent. Therefore, the person experiences the sensation of bladder fullness but cannot voluntarily inhibit micturition (Dittmar, 1989).

Urinary incontinence and dementia often coexist (Skelly & Flint, 1995). As the areas of the cerebral cortex become more affected by dementia, there is a corresponding decline in function of the body part under the control of the affected area. As the disease progresses, the individual with dementia also loses the ability to recognize the sensation of bladder fullness, remember the location of the toilet, and communicate the need to use the toilet. People with dementia may also develop transient incontinence due to non-neurogenic causes.

Hyper-reflexic responses of the detrusor to filling of urine occur frequently in demyelinating diseases such as multiple sclerosis. In these cases the bladder is spastic, attempting to empty urine often without synchronization with the external sphincter function, resulting in frequent, small voidings. This is known as detrusor sphincter dyssynergia (DSD) (Fantl et al., 1996).

If the spinal cord is totally severed above the sacral reflex center as a result of an accident or surgery, or is occluded by a lesion, no sensory signals are received by the cortex and, consequently, no inhibitory signals are sent to the bladder. Emptying of the bladder relies solely on the sacral reflex center. The contractions of the detrusor are less efficient than those under cortical control and, of course, the emptying is completely involuntary and less efficient.

Sacral Spinal Lesions

Injuries or diseases that interfere with the sacral spinal cord functioning are additional neurological causes of incontinence. Examples include vascular diseases, peripheral nerve lesions, diabetes mellitus, tabes dorsalis, alcoholic neuropathy, and trauma from surgery or accidents to the sacral region of the spine.

If the sensory input from the bladder (afferent nerve pathways) is disrupted, as in diabetes mellitus, tabes dorsalis, alcoholic neuropathy, or trauma, conscious control over micturition and efficient detrusor contraction are lost. The bladder becomes flaccid, or atonic, holding large amounts of urine until overflow incontinence occurs.

Increased Afferent Loop Stimulation

The bladder is also a site of neurological activity. Stretch receptors and autonomic nerve endings are located within the bladder walls. In the presence of disease or obstruction such as urinary tract infection, neoplasm, enlarged prostate, organ prolapse, fecal impaction, or urethral stricture, abnormally rapid transmission and reception of sensory impulses can cause defective, uninhibited contractions resulting in urge incontinence.

The neurological component of micturition is complex and not completely understood. Specific areas of control and the relationship with urinary tract function require more investigation by researchers before definitive statements about specific causal relationships can be made. It can be stated, however, that a neurological disruption at any point of the micturition cycle, if severe enough, can cause overflow or urge incontinence in any individual.

ENVIRONMENTAL FACTORS

Environmental factors associated with urinary incontinence are factors external to the older adult that, acting alone or in combination with physical or cognitive impairments, cause incontinence. There is evidence that factors (e.g., impaired mobility) outside the anatomical structures involved in micturition play a role in the prevalence of incontinence (Yu et al., 1990). Psychological factors contributing to incontinence are discussed in detail in Chapter 6.

Environmental factors associated with incontinence include medications (see Exhibit 3–6), location of the bathroom, appropriateness of the toilet facilities, provisions for privacy and safety, and types of garments.

Medications

Diuretics

The combination of impaired mobility and fast-acting diuretics, such as furosemide, can cause or exacerbate urinary incontinence in older adults. Diuretics increase urine production and the frequency of voiding (Shimp, Wells, Brink, Diokno, & Gillis, 1988). At times this can overwhelm the person's ability to delay voiding until the toilet is reached. In this situation the individual cannot reach toilet facilities in time and has an "accident."

Sedative Hypnotics

Excessive sedation and strong hypnotics can also contribute to incontinence by preventing the older adult from awakening in time to maneuver to the toilet. Sedative hypnotics can also delay the conscious perception of the need to void until the individual has insufficient time between awareness of the need to void and the involuntary emptying of urine from the bladder. Also, confusion and disorientation are serious side effects of many sedatives and hypnotics. A state of confusion and disorientation places the older adult at high risk for incontinence.

Anticholinergic Medications

Medications with anticholinergic action contribute to the retention of urine, possibly leading to overflow incontinence (see Table 3–2). Individuals with compromised bladder outlets, such as men with benign prostatic hyperplasia, are at risk of developing overflow incontinence due to the potential side effect of urinary retention (Zawada, 1985). Nurses and other health care providers should consult with a pharmacist if they are uncertain of the potential action or side effect of any medication before administering it.

Exhibit 3-6 Medications That Can Affect Continence

Medication Type or Class	Effect on Urine Control
Diuretics	Frequent and large bladder volume may overwhelm the ability to reach the bathroom in time.
Sedative hypnotics	Depress sensorium and ability to discern the need to empty the bladder. May cause excessive muscle relaxation.
Anticholinergics (includes antipsychotics and antidepressants)	Retain urine by inhibiting bladder contractibility and may cause overflow incontinence in susceptible individuals, e.g., men with benign prostatic hyperplasia.
Narcotics	Depress sensorium and ability to discern the need to empty the bladder. Cause fecal impaction, resulting in pressure on the bladder, and may decrease bladder capacity.
Parkinson's disease medication (except Sinemet and deprenyl)	May cause dribbling via decreased sphincter strength.
Disopyramide	Anticholinergic properties may lead to retention and overflow incontinence.
Antispasmodics	May cause excessive muscular relaxation and sphincter incompetency.
Antihistamines	May cause urinary retention, leading to overflow incontinence.
Calcium channel blockers	Reduce detrusor contractions and may lead to urinary retention and overflow incontinence.
Drugs that affect the sympathetic nervous system	Alpha-blockers may relax the smooth muscle of the sphincter and decrease urethral pressure and increase bladder emptying. Alpha-stimulants may increase urethral closure pressure and lead to urinary retention.

Source: Reprinted from Palmer, M., Basic Assessment and Management of Urinary Incontinence in Nursing Homes, Level I, *Nurse Practitioner Forum,* Vol. 5, No. 3, p. 154, with permission of W.B. Saunders, © 1994.

Table 3–2 Examples of Medications with Urinary Retention As a Side Effect*

Type	Generic Name	Brand Name
Antidepressants	Amitriptyline hydrochloride	Elavil
	Desipramine hydrochloride	Norpramin
	Doxepin hydrochloride	Sinequan
	Fluoxetine hydrochloride	Prozac
	Imipramine pamoate	Tofranil-PM
	Nortriptyline hydrochloride	Pamelor
Antihistamines	Brompheniramine maleate	Dimetane
	Chlorpheniramine maleate	Many medications
	Diphenhydramine hydrochloride	Benadryl
	Meclizine hydrochloride	Antivert
	Pheniramine maleate	Many medications
	Pseudoephedrine hydrochloride	Many medications
	Pyrilamine maleate	Many medications
Anti-Parkinson disease	Amantadine hydrochloride	Symmetrel
	Benztropine mesylate	Cogentin
	Bromocriptine mesylate	Parlodel
	Hyoscyamine sulfate	Levsin Cystospaz-M
	Orphenadrine citrate	Norflex
	Procyclidine hydrochloride	Kemadrin
	Trihexyphenidyl hydrochloride	Artane
	Levdopa and carbidopa	Sinemet
Belladonna alkaloids	Atropine sulfate	Donnagel
	Scopolamine hydrobromide	Donnatal
Phenothiazines	Chlorpromazine hydrochloride	Thorazine
	Perphenazine	Trilafon
	Prochlorperazine	Compazine
	Thioridazine hydrochloride	Mellaril
	Trifluoperazine hydrochloride	Stelazine

*This list is not inclusive. Consult a pharmacist to determine whether a medication has urinary retention as a side effect before administration.

Alcohol

Alcohol has several beneficial effects for older adults (Atkinson, Ganzini, & Bernstein, 1991). Appetite enhancement, vasodilatation, and anxiety reduction are a few examples. However, some side effects can contribute to the development of incontinence. Alcohol has a profound sedative effect. Therefore, the conscious awareness of the need to void may be compromised. The diuretic effect causes the body to produce a larger volume of urine that the individual may not be able to accommodate. Incontinence can also be caused by the ingestion of alcohol to the point of impaired mobility and inebriation.

Toilet Facilities

Although an individual may successfully reach the toilet facilities, the height of the commode and the space to maneuver walkers and canes can play an important role in the development of incontinence. The provision for privacy is another important consideration. Stalls without doors and lack of privacy can discourage an older adult from using the toilet facilities. Cleanliness, poor lighting in bathrooms, and inadequate staff assistance to use the toilet can also serve as a deterrent and lessen an older adult's attempts to use the facilities (Jirovec, Brink, & Wells, 1988).

One of the greatest fears of older adults is falling. Falling when attempting to meet elimination needs is a serious problem (Garcia et al., 1988). In some cases, toilet facilities that are perceived as being unsafe by an older adult will not be used. Attempts at makeshift commodes and urinals will be made, often further risking the safety of the older adult. Nighttime incontinence can occur if the bed is too high for an older adult to get into and out of safely without assistance. In institutions, the availability of nursing staff, especially during the night, can be a factor in the development of incontinence. Some older adults who are ambulatory during the day may not be able to walk in bare feet or slippers at night. Stooping to put on supportive shoes may increase pressure on the bladder and delay voiding beyond the ability to retain urine. Thus the seemingly simple act of going to the toilet can require a great deal of physical energy and agility. When these requirements exceed the physical capabilities of the older adult the consequence may be urinary incontinence.

Clothing

Clothing items that are difficult or time consuming to remove can contribute to the development of incontinence. The potent combination of arthritic hands attempting to pull down a zipper or open a button and an increased urgency to void caused by a diuretic places the older adult at high risk for becoming incontinent. Tight undergarments and constricting girdles can exert increased pressure on the bladder. Clothing options to promote independence and continence are discussed in Chapter 8.

CONCLUSION

In many cases, the cause of incontinence is a combination of several factors. Many normal changes with age predispose the older adult to be at risk for developing incontinence. A change in environment, an acute illness that limits mobility or fatigues the older adult, or a urinary tract infection that increases urgency can tip the delicate balance of continent urinary function toward transient incontinence. If the transient incontinence is complacently accepted by the older adult and caregiver, the eventual result may well be established incontinence.

REFERENCES

Appell, R. (1994). Pathogenesis and medical management of benign prostatic hyperplasia. *Seminars in Nephrology, 14*, 531–543.

Atkinson, R., Ganzini, L., & Bernstein, M. (1991). Alcohol and substance-use disorders in the elderly. In J. Birren, R. Sloane, & G. Cohen (Eds.), *Handbook of mental health and aging.* New York: Academic Press.

Barry, M. (1993). Epidemiology and natural history of benign prostatic hyperplasia. In H. Lepor & R. Lawson (Eds.), *Prostate disease.* Philadelphia: Saunders.

Bump, R., Bo, K., Brubaker, L., DeLancey, J., Klarskov, P., Shull, B., & Smith, A. (1995). The standardisation of terminology of female pelvic organ prolapse and pelvic floor dysfunction. *International Continence Society Committee on Standardisation of Terminology,* 1–12.

Clinical Practice Guideline Panel. (1994). *Clinical practice guideline: Benign prostatic hyperplasia: Diagnosis and treatment* (AHCPR Pub. No. 94-0582). Rockville, MD: Agency for Health Care Policy and Research, Public Health Service, U.S. Department of Health and Human Services.

Diokno, A., Brock, B., Brown, M., & Herzog, R. (1986). Prevalence of urinary incontinence and other urological symptoms in the noninstitutionalized elderly. *Journal of Urology, 136*, 1022–1025.

Dittmar, S. (1989). *Rehabilitation nursing: Process and application.* St. Louis: Mosby.

Fantl, A., Cardozo, L., McClish, D., & the Hormones and Urogenital Therapy Committee. (1994). Estrogen therapy in the management of urinary incontinence in postmenopausal women: A meta-analysis: First report of the hormones and urogenital therapy committee. *Obstetrics and Gynecology, 83*, 12–18.

Fantl, J.A., Newman, D.K., & Colling, J. et al. (1996). *Urinary incontinence in adults: Acute and chronic management. Clinical practice guideline no. 2, 1996 update.* (AHCPR Pub. No. 96-0692). Rockville, MD: Agency for Health Care Policy and Research, Public Health Service, U.S. Department of Health and Human Services.

Garcia, R., Cruz, M., Reed, M., Taylor, P., Sloan, G., & Beran, N. (1988). Relationship between falls and patient attempts to satisfy elimination needs. *Nursing Management, 19*(7), 80V–80X.

Harris, T. (1986). Aging in the eighties: Prevalence and impact of urinary problems in individuals age 65 years and over. *NCHS Advance Data* (DHHS Publication No. 86-1250, pp. 1–8). Hyattsville, MD: U.S. Department of Health and Human Services.

Herzog, A., Fultz, N., Brock, B., Brown, M., & Diokno, A. (1988). Urinary incontinence and psychological distress among older adults. *Psychology and Aging, 3*, 115–121.

Hing, E., & Sekscenski, E. (1986). Use of health care-nursing home care. *NCHS Analytical and Epidemiological Series 3, No. 25,* 71–75.

Jirovec, M., Brink, C., & Wells, T. (1988). Nursing assessment in the inpatient geriatric population. *Nursing Clinics of North America, 23,* 219–230.

Massachusetts Medical Society. (1991). Urinary incontinence among hospitalized persons aged 65 years and older—United States, 1984–1987. *Morbidity and Mortality Weekly Reports, 40,* 433–436.

Mohide, E., Pringle, D., Robertson, D., & Chambers, L. (1988). Prevalence of urinary incontinence in patients receiving home care services. *Canadian Medical Association Journal, 139,* 953–956.

Motola, J., & Badlani, G. (1990). Cerebrovascular accidents. Urological effects and management. *Clinics in Geriatric Medicine, 6,* 55–68.

Nygaard, I., Thompson, F., Svengalis, S., & Albright, J. (1994). Urinary incontinence in elite nulliparous athletes. *Obstetrics and Gynecology, 84,* 183–187.

Ouslander, J., & Fowler, E. (1985). Management of urinary incontinence in Veterans Administration nursing homes. *Journal of the American Geriatrics Society, 33,* 33–40.

Ouslander, J., Kane, R., & Abrass, I. (1982). Urinary incontinence in elderly nursing home patients. *Journal of the American Medical Association, 248,* 1194–1198.

Palmer, M., Bone, L., Fahey, M., Mamon, J., & Steinwachs, D. (1992). Detecting urinary incontinence in older adults during hospitalization. *Applied Nursing Research, 5,* 1–7.

Palmer, M., German, P., & Ouslander, J. (1991). Risk factors for urinary incontinence one year after nursing home admission. *Research in Nursing and Health, 14,* 405–412.

Raz, S. (1978). Pathophysiology of male incontinence. *Urologic Clinics of North America, 5,* 295–304.

Rekers, H., Drogendijk, A., Valkenburg, H., & Riphagen, F. (1992). The menopause, urinary incontinence and other symptoms of the genito-urinary tract. *Maturitas, 15,* 101–111.

Resnick, N., & Yalla, S. (1987a). Aging and its effect on the bladder. *Seminars in Urology, 5*(2), 82–86.

Resnick, N., & Yalla, S. (1987b). Detrusor hyperactivity with impaired contractile function. *Journal of the American Medical Association, 257,* 3076–3081.

Resnick, N., & Yalla, S. (1992). Evaluation and medical management of urinary incontinence. In P. Walsh, A. Retisk, T. Stamey, & E. Vaughan (Eds.), *Campbell's urology* (6th ed.). Philadelphia: Saunders.

Shimp, L., Wells, T., Brink, C., Diokno, C., & Gillis, G. (1988, October). Relationship between drug use and urinary incontinence in elderly women. *Drug Intelligence and Clinical Pharmacy, 22,* 786–787.

Shortlife, L., & Stamey, T. (1986). Urinary incontinence in the female. In P. Walsh, R. Gittes, P. Perlmutter, & T. Stamey (Eds.), *Campbell's urology* (5th ed., Vol. 3). Philadelphia: Saunders.

Sier, H., Ouslander, J., Orzeck, S. (1987). Urinary incontinence among geriatric patients in an acute-care hospital. *Journal of the American Medical Association, 257,* 1767–1771.

Skelly, J., & Flint, A. (1995). Urinary incontinence associated with dementia. *Journal of the American Geriatrics Society, 43,* 286–294.

Sullivan, D., & Lindsay, R. (1984). Urinary incontinence in the geriatric population of an acute care hospital. *Journal of the American Geriatrics Society, 31,* 694–697.

Tinetti, M., Inouye, S., Gill, T., & Doucette, J. (1995). Shared risk factors for falls, incontinence, and functional dependence. *Journal of the American Medical Association, 273,* 1348–1353.

Ulmsten, U. (1995). On urogenital ageing. *Maturitas, 21*, 163–169.

Versi, E. (1990). Incontinence in the climacteric. *Clinical Obstetrics and Gynecology, 33*, 392–398.

Wall, L., Norton, P., & DeLancey, J. (1993). Prolapse and the lower urinary tract. In L. Wall, P. Norton, & J. DeLancey (Eds.), *Practical urogynecology*. Baltimore: Williams & Wilkins.

Wein, A. (1993). Criteria for assessing outcome following intervention for benign prostatic hyperplasia. In H. Lepor & R. Lawson (Eds.), *Prostate disease*. Philadelphia: Saunders.

Wetle, T., Scherr, P., Branch, L., Resnick, N., Harris, T., Evans, D., & Taylor, J. (1995). Difficulty with holding urine among older persons in a geographically defined community: Prevalence and correlates. *Journal of the American Geriatrics Society, 43*, 349–355.

Yu, L., Rohner, T., Kaltreider, L., Hu, T., Igou, J., & Dennis, P. (1990). Profile of urinary incontinent elderly in long-term care institutions. *Journal of the American Geriatrics Society, 38*, 433–439.

Zawada, E. (1985). Voiding problems in the elderly: Functional disorders of the lower urinary tract. In E. Zawada & D. Sica (Eds.), *Geriatric nephrology and urology*. Littleton, MA: PSG Publishing.

CHAPTER

4

Assessment

Urinary incontinence has subjective and objective manifestations (see Exhibit 4–1). Increasingly, health care providers recognize that incontinence is a highly treatable condition. Most incontinence can be improved or cured (Fantl, Newman, & Colling et al., 1996).

However, before treatment options are implemented, a thorough assessment that includes a detailed history, a physical and functional assessment, and urinalysis must be conducted. The approach to the assessment of incontinence, regardless of the health care setting, generally is the same. Screening and assessment for potentially reversible or transient causes and simple urodynamic testing occur first. More sophisticated testing occurs if incontinence does not improve or worsens. However, if in the initial assessment there is evidence of serious urogenital or neurological disease or damage, prompt treatment is essential.

This chapter provides an overview of the assessment process for transient and established incontinence. The focus is on assessment of incontinence in the older adult. Discussion of complex urodynamic testing is beyond the scope of this book; however, comprehensive history taking, physical examination, and simple urodynamic testing are discussed.

NURSING'S ROLE

Nurses play a central role in the assessment of incontinence. Historically, nurses have enjoyed a special relationship with their patients. Not only do nurses have close physical contact to assess physiologic parameters, change dressings, and perform other nursing functions, but they also develop empathetic, caring relationships that provide and promote the emotional well-being of their patients. The older adult with urinary incontinence may be more willing to discuss the symptoms

Exhibit 4–1 Manifestations of Urinary Incontinence

	Subjective	Objective
Stress	Report of small amount of urine loss with a cough, sneeze, laugh, change of position; sensation of heaviness in pelvic area	Leaking of urine with standing and/or lying stress test; hypermobility of urethra during voiding cystometrogram; evidence of weak vaginal tone, cystocele, atrophic vaginitis, or sphincter incompetence during pelvic exam
Urge	Report of need to void comes on too fast to get to toilet; loss of large amount of urine; frequent voiding; loss of urine at sound of water running or when waiting for access to a public toilet	Evidence of urinary tract infection, inflammation of bladder wall; uninhibited bladder contractions on cystometrogram; evidence of neurological lesion in cerebral cortex; deconditioned micturition reflex during physical exam
Overflow	Report of incomplete emptying of the bladder; dribbling of urine; painful abdomen; unaware of urine loss	Palpable bladder during abdominal exam; large amount of urine in bladder after voiding; evidence of outlet obstruction (i.e., enlarged prostate palpated during rectal exam)
Functional	Report of inability to get to bathroom on time; inability to position for toileting without assistance; lack of convenient access to toilet	No incontinence when access to toilet or assistance to toilet is available; evidence of impaired mobility, manual dexterity, communication, or cognitive skills; normal functioning of urinary tract during urodynamic testing

Source: Reprinted from Palmer, M., Urinary Incontinence in *Pathophysiological Phenomena in Nursing*, 2nd ed., by V. Carrieri-Kohlman, A. Lindsay and C. West, p. 231, with permission of W.B. Saunders, © 1993.

and impact of urinary incontinence with a nurse than with other health care professionals because of the perceived empathy and trustworthiness of the nurse. The atmosphere of competence and empathy that the nurse creates can help the older adult to disclose information about urinary incontinence.

The nursing perspective of the client is unique. The nurse takes a comprehensive approach in assessing not only the client but the environment surrounding the client. This approach is reflected in the questions asked during the nursing history (see Exhibit 4–2).

Exhibit 4–2 Continence Assessment Form

Name:_____ Age:_____

General Health
Mini-mental state examination score: _____
Other medical conditions: _____
Living arrangements: _____
Current medications: _____
Special diet: _____
Fluid intake (include restrictions): _____
History of previous surgeries (include urogenital, spinal surgeries):
_____
History of cerebrovascular accident or head trauma: _____
How do you rate your health?   Poor   Fair   Good   Excellent

Continence Status
How many times do you pass your urine in one day? _____
How many continent voids? _____ How many incontinent voids? _____
How much urine loss occurs with an incontinent void? _____
Do you experience urine loss before reaching the toilet? _____
How often? _____
When does the urine loss most occur (day/night/both)? _____
Do you leak urine without knowing it? _____
Do you leak urine when you cough, sneeze, laugh, change positions? _____
Do you leak urine at night while you sleep? _____
How long have you had a problem with urine control? _____
Have you ever consulted a health care provider about a urine control problem?
_____
What was done to treat it? _____

Environmental Assessment
How far do you walk to the bathroom where you live? _____
Do you need to go upstairs? _____ Is this a problem for you? _____
Do you have difficulty in getting to the bathroom at night? _____
Do you have difficulty in getting up from the toilet? _____
Do you have difficulty in removing or fastening clothing? _____
How much fluid do you drink during the day? _____
Do you drink fluids in the evening? _____ What kind? _____ How much? _____
Do you drink alcohol? _____ How much? _____
Do you drink caffeinated coffee, tea, or sodas? _____
Amount and frequency _____
Do you smoke? _____ How much? _____ For how long? _____
Do you use aspartame as a sweetener? _____ Do you take fluid pills (diuretics)? _____
Do you have diabetes mellitus? _____ How long have you been diagnosed? _____
How is it controlled? _____ What was your last blood sugar level? _____
Do you experience constipation? _____ Fecal impactions? _____

continues

Exhibit 4–2 continued

Neurological History
How long can you delay emptying your bladder after feeling the need to void? _____
Can you tell when your bladder is full? _____
Do you empty your bladder completely when you void? _____
When voiding, do you know when the urine flow starts? _____ Stops? _____

Questions for Women
What is the date of your last menses? _____
Have you ever been pregnant? _____ Given birth? _____
Were forceps used during the delivery(s)? _____
Have you ever been given hormone replacement therapy? _____
Did you have any side effects? _____
Are you undergoing hormone replacement therapy now? _____
Have you ever had surgery for prolapse of the uterus? _____ bladder? _____ rectum? _____
Have you had a hysterectomy? _____ Have you had colon surgery? _____
Do you use panty liners, sanitary napkins, tissue, disposable briefs, or any other absorbent material for urine control? _____
Does urine escape from you when you raise or lower yourself in a chair? _____
Is it difficult to stop the urine once it starts flowing? _____
Do you leak urine when you are nervous or excited? _____
Do you wear a girdle? _____

Questions for Men
When was your last rectal exam? _____ Results? _____
When was your last prostate-specific antigen test? _____ Results? _____
How often do you get up at night to void? _____
Do you have difficulty in starting to void? _____
Is your stream of urine less forceful than it used to be? _____
Have you noticed blood in your urine? _____
Does your bladder feel empty after you finish voiding? _____
Have you had a urinary tract infection recently? _____
Do you have to strain to empty your bladder? _____

History of Urinary Tract Infections
Do you feel pain or burning when you urinate? _____
Do you have any pain in your lower back or your sides? _____
Is your urine cloudy? _____ What is the color of your urine? _____
How often do you pass urine? _____ During the day? _____ At night? _____
How do you wipe yourself after voiding? (front to back?) _____
How long can you wait after you feel the need to void? _____
Does it feel like you empty your bladder completely? _____
Have you ever had a urinary tract infection? _____ When? _____
How was it treated? _____

continues

Exhibit 4-2 continued

Informational Needs
What do you think is wrong? _____
What do you want done about the urine control problem now? _____
How do you manage it now? _____
Has incontinence changed the way you live your life? _____
Do you go out for social activities? _____
What do you do to prevent or control urine leakage? _____
Do you feel that you need more information about treating urine control loss? _____
What kind of information would be useful to you? _____

Additional Information

Because incontinence is a complex condition, the interprofessional approach is important as assessment proceeds and treatment options are discussed. The incontinent person benefits from this approach because the sharing of information and resources among health care providers knowledgeable about incontinence helps them to view the individual in a holistic manner.

ASSESSMENT IN THE LONG-TERM CARE SETTING

The basic assessment process of incontinence in long-term care facilities has been designed in order for the nurse to perform it at the bedside with other health care providers (e.g., physicians, social workers, physical therapists) as consultants. Since 1990, the Minimum Data Set (MDS), a standardized screening and assessment form, has been completed on all residents at admission, quarterly, and when a significant change in medical status occurs. The continence section of the MDS is displayed in Exhibit 4-3.

When a resident is found to be incontinent or has an indwelling catheter, further assessment using the Resident Assessment Profile (RAP) is required. The RAP provides a rapid, yet comprehensive problem-solving approach to detect the causes of incontinence. The first part of the RAP is used to detect transient or potentially reversible causes of incontinence (Palmer, 1994). The second part of the RAP is used if incontinence persists or worsens after the preliminary assessment and treatment.

52 URINARY CONTINENCE

Exhibit 4–3 Minimum Data Set (MDS) Section H, Continence

SECTION H. CONTINENCE IN LAST 14 DAYS

1. CONTINENCE SELF-CONTROL CATEGORIES
   (Code for resident's performance over all shifts.)
   0. CONTINENT—Complete control (includes use of indwelling urinary catheter or ostomy device that does not leak urine or stool)
   1. USUALLY CONTINENT—BLADDER, incontinent episodes once a week or less; BOWEL, less than weekly
   2. OCCASIONALLY INCONTINENT—BLADDER, 2 or more times a week but not daily; BOWEL, once a week
   3. FREQUENTLY INCONTINENT—BLADDER, tended to be incontinent daily, but some control present (e.g, on day shift); BOWEL, 2–3 times a week
   4. INCONTINENT—Had inadequate control. BLADDER, multiple daily episodes; BOWEL, all (or almost all) of the time

   a. **BOWEL CONTINENCE** — Control of bowel movement, with appliance or bowel continence programs, if employed

   b. **BLADDER CONTINENCE** — Control of urinary bladder function (if dribbles, volume insufficient to soak through underpants), with appliances (e.g., Foley) or continence programs, if employed

2. **BOWEL ELIMINATION PATTERN**

Bowel elimination pattern regular—at least one movement every three days	a.	Diarrhea	c.	
		Fecal impaction	d.	
Constipation	b.	NONE OF ABOVE	e.	

3. **APPLIANCES AND PROGRAMS**

Any scheduled toileting plan	a.	Did not use toilet room/commode/urinal	f.	
Bladder retraining program	b.	Pads/briefs used	g.	
External (condom) catheter	c.	Enemas/irrigation	h.	
Indwelling catheter	d.	Ostomy present	i.	
Intermittent catheter	e.	NONE OF ABOVE	j.	

4. **CHANGE IN URINARY CONTINENCE** — Resident's urinary continence has changed as compared to status of **90 days ago** (or since last assessment if less than 90 days)
   0. No change   1. Improved   2. Deteriorated

Source: Reprinted from *Long-Term Care Facility Assessment Instrument (RAI) User's Manual, Version 2.0,* by J. Morris, K. Murphy, and S. Nonemaker, p. B-6, with permission of the Health Care Financing Administration, © 1995.

The nurse elicits information from the resident, caregiver, medical record, and other sources about the presence of the conditions or factors that could affect continence. At all times, however, the resident is the center of the assessment, whose right to privacy and dignity must be preserved.

Mobility

The inability to ambulate and use the toilet independently can influence the development and presence of incontinence. Mobility can be assessed by direct observation, use of standardized tests, and consultation with physical therapists. Assessing toileting skills can be conducted by using POTTI (performance on timed toileting instrument). This instrument consists of five tasks that simulate toileting. They include walking or moving 15 feet; transferring to a commode; unfastening a hook; unzipping a zipper; and pulling down a garment (Ouslander et al., 1987).

Medications

All medications and the timing of their administration should be assessed for their effects on continence. Medications with a diuretic, muscle relaxant, urinary retention, or sedation effect should be carefully evaluated for need of their continued use and their effect on continence (see Exhibit 3–6 and Table 3–2).

Delirium

The presence of delirium, a sudden change in sensorium, should be carefully assessed. Often delirium is the first sign of infection (Fox, 1988). Addition or changes in medications, changes in fluid and electrolyte balance, presence of pain, fecal impaction, and sleep deprivation are other causes of delirium in older adults. The underlying cause of delirium must be ascertained.

Medical Conditions

Medical conditions such as diabetes mellitus, congestive heart failure (CHF), urinary tract infections (UTIs), fecal impaction, and depression can cause or make existing incontinence worse. Polyuria is an acute symptom of diabetes mellitus. With the body's attempt to rid the body of excess glucose, diuresis results and increases the risk of overwhelming the bladder with the excess fluid volume. Also, a long-term consequence of diabetes mellitus is peripheral neuropathy, a lower neuron disruption, leading to incomplete emptying of the bladder.

In individuals with CHF, fluid mobilization may occur at night while there is less stress on the heart. As diuresis occurs, the individual may have incontinent episodes due to the excessive volume of urine, inability to wake in time, and inability to reach the toilet in time. Medications used in the treatment of CHF, especially diuretics, can cause incontinence by increasing urine volume.

McGeer et al. (1991) recommend that identification of symptomatic urinary tract infections in nursing home residents include at least three of the classic signs and symptoms (see Exhibit 4–4). Other signs and symptoms may include altered mental status, loss of appetite, lethargy, and changes in ability to perform activities of daily living (ADLs) (Schultz & Gambert, 1991), although there is little research available indicating that these latter symptoms are indicative of a urinary infection (Nicolle, 1993). A microscopic examination of the urine for bacteria and white blood cells, a dipstick test for the presence of leukocyte esterase and nitrite, and a urine culture are objective measures of bacteriuria.

Obtaining a sterile specimen, without catheterization, is possible with individuals who are unable to collect the specimen independently (Ouslander, Schapira, & Schnelle, 1995; Brazier & Palmer, 1995). Using information about the person's voiding habits, getting assistance from others, and applying sterile external collection devices are some of the important steps. Many institutionalized older adults have chronic bacteriuria that presents with no clinical symp-

---

Exhibit 4–4 Signs and Symptoms of Urinary Tract Infections

Classic Signs and Symptoms
 Fever or chills
 Flank, lower back, suprapubic pain
 Burning on urination
 Dysuria
 Frequency
 Urgency
 Pyuria
 Microscopic hematuria
Possible Signs and Symptoms
 Delirium or altered mental status
 Decline in ability to perform ADLs
 Lethargy
 Decreased appetite

toms. Generally chronic asymptomatic bacteriuria is left untreated (Kane, Ouslander, & Abrass, 1994).

Depression

Depression is prevalent in the older population (Callahan, Hui, Nienaber, Musick, & Tierney, 1994). Its presence may affect an older person's continence (Wyman, 1988). Some signs of depression include weight loss or gain, motor retardation or agitation, sad mood for at least 2 weeks, inability to enjoy activities, fatigue, thoughts of suicide, and sleep disruptions (Koenig & Blazer, 1991). There are several screening tools that can help detect the presence of depression, such as the CES-D (Radloff, 1977). Some medications may cause depression in older adults. The first step in treatment, however, is detecting and reporting depression to a health care provider knowledgeable in treating affective disorders in older adults. If detected and reported, depression can be effectively treated.

Toilet Facilities

The environment should be assessed as well; inaccessibility of the toilet can cause incontinence. Even though a resident may live in a semiprivate room with its own bathroom, most daytime hours may be spent in activities rooms or common rooms where access to the toilet is limited. Therefore, the nurse needs to determine toilet accessibility given the daily social calendar, staffing patterns, and overall physical layout of the nursing unit.

Further Assessment

If incontinence persists or becomes worse, further assessment is required. Women residents should be physically examined for signs of urethritis, vaginitis, and prolapse. Postvoid residual urine volume should be obtained to determine the effectiveness of bladder emptying. A noninvasive reliable method using a portable ultrasound device is available (Ouslander et al., 1994). Selection of the right size speculum for the examination is important. Prior to inserting the speculum, the examiner should assess the vaginal mucosa and determine the depth of the vagina (Brazier, 1994). One of the most commonly used specula is the Graves speculum. It has curved blades that vary in length from 3.5 to 5 inches and in width from 0.75 to 0.125 inch. The larger speculum should be used for women who have had multiple births, have prolapsed anterior vaginal walls, or are obese (Varney, 1987). Other specula are available as well. The Pederson specula are as long as the Graves specula but have narrower blades and are appropriate for nulliparous women. A virginal speculum has narrow and short blades and is appropriate for sexually inactive women (Varney, 1987).

Having a good light source for the examination is critical. A free-standing lamp with a 150-W bulb positioned over the shoulder of the examiner is an excellent source of light. A headlamp sold in camping catalogues is a very effective and inexpensive device that can be used in any setting where an examination is to be performed. The nurse or health care provider conducting the exam should be skilled at putting the woman at ease for the examination, using techniques such as breathing relaxation exercises or imagery. Ideally the woman needs to be placed in the lithotomy position for the pelvic examination. However, this position can be painful for a woman with arthritic hips or a history of hip surgery. In this case, the examination can be performed while the woman lies on her side with the top leg flexed and crossed over the leg resting on the bed (Kinney, Blount, & Dowell, 1980). A pillow should be placed under her head and she should be draped at all times.

Signs of urethritis and vaginitis include dry, thin, reddened tissue with or without discharge and complaints of itching or pain. Presence of a pelvic prolapse can be assessed by asking the woman to bear down and by placing one blade of the speculum into the vagina, pressing it against the anterior vaginal wall and then the posterior vaginal wall (Brazier, 1994).

Men should be assessed for signs and symptoms of benign prostatic hyperplasia (see Exhibit 4–5).

Complaints of bladder pain and evidence of hematuria could indicate a serious underlying pathology, e.g., bladder cancer or renal stone. A physician referral is essential.

The original Clinical Practice Guideline Panel (1992a) provided an algorithm for the assessment of incontinence in nursing home residents (see Figure 4–1).

ASSESSMENT OF NONINSTITUTIONALIZED OLDER ADULTS

History

The questions asked during the history taking can seem invasive and embarrassing to the affected adult. Some of the tests on physical examination can be embarrassing and uncomfortable. It is particularly important to remember that the older adult's reaction time in responding to questions may be slower than a younger adult's, and a lengthy assessment interview can easily be tiring. A focused review of systems is outlined in Exhibit 4–6.

Older Adults' Responses to Assessment

Initially the health care provider should be prepared for older adults to be reluctant to talk about incontinent behavior. The majority of incontinent older

Exhibit 4–5 The American Urological Association (AUA) Symptom Index

Question	Not at All	Less Than 1 Time in 5	Less Than Half the Time	About Half the Time	More Than Half the Time	Almost Always
1. During the last month or so, how often have you had a sensation of not emptying your bladder completely after you finished urinating?	0	1	2	3	4	5
2. During the last month or so, how often have you had to urinate again less than 2 hours after you finished urinating?	0	1	2	3	4	5
3. During the last month or so, how often have you found you stopped and started again several times when you urinated?	0	1	2	3	4	5
4. During the last month or so, how often have you found it difficult to postpone urination?	0	1	2	3	4	5
5. During the last month or so, how often have you had a weak urinary stream?	0	1	2	3	4	5
6. During the last month or so, how often have you had to push or strain to begin urination?	0	1	2	3	4	5

	None	1 Time	2 Times	3 Times	4 Times	5 or More Times
7. During the last month, how many times did you most typically get up to urinate from the time you went to bed at night until the time you got up in the morning?	0	1	2	3	4	5

AUA symptom score = sum of questions 1 to 7.

Source: Reprinted from Barry, M. et al., The AUA Symptom Index for Benign Prostatic Hyperplasia, *Journal of Urology*, Vol. 148, pp. 1549–1557, with permission of Williams & Wilkins, © 1992.

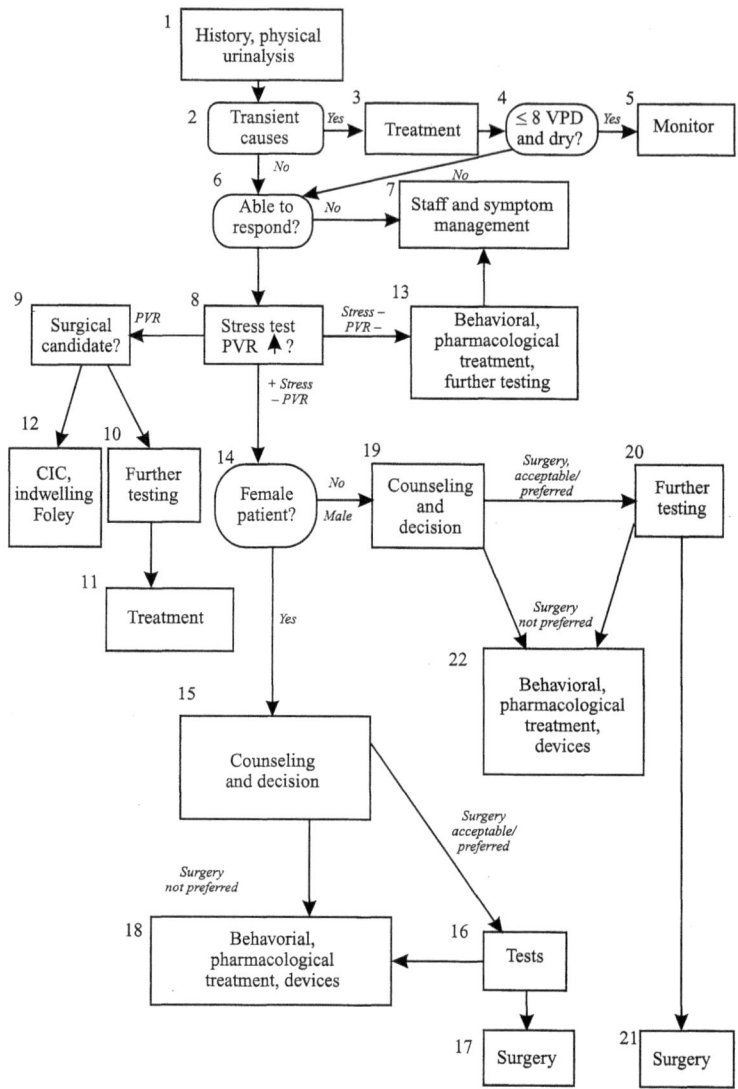

VPD, voids per day; PVR, postvoid residual; CIC, clean intermittent catheterization

Figure 4–1 Algorithm for Assessment of Nursing Home/Frail Elderly Stress/Urge/Other Incontinence. *Source:* Reprinted from Clinical Practice Guideline Panel, *Clinical Practice Guideline: Urinary Incontinence in Adults,* p. 85, Agency for Health Care Policy and Research, U.S. Department of Health and Human Services, Publication No. 92-0038, 1992.

Exhibit 4–6 Focused Review of Systems

I. Urological system
   A. Urinary tract infection
      1. Lower urinary tract infection (cystitis)
      2. Upper urinary tract infection (pyelonephritis)
      3. History of vesicoureteral reflux
   B. Urinary tract tumors and stones
   C. Renal insufficiency
   D. Other urinary tract problems
II. Neurological system
   A. General indicators of dysfunction (motor-sensory loss)
   B. Central nervous system
      1. Lesions
         a. Tumor
         b. Stroke
         c. Multiple sclerosis
         d. Others
      2. Organic diseases
         a. Alzheimer's disease
         b. Others
      3. Trauma
      4. Surgical procedures
   C. Spinal cord
      1. Injury
         a. Vertebral level
         b. Extent of involvement
      2. Lesions and conditions
         a. Multiple sclerosis
         b. Transverse myelitis
         c. Others
   D. Peripheral nervous system
      1. Back conditions and treatments
      2. Peripheral neuropathy
         a. Symptoms
         b. Associated medical conditions
            (1) Diabetes mellitus
            (2) Others
III. Reproductive system
   A. Female
      1. Number of vaginal deliveries
      2. Obstetrical complications or difficult deliveries
      3. Gynecologic conditions
         a. Vaginitis
         b. Sexually transmitted diseases
         c. Others

continues

Exhibit 4–6 continued

          4. Premenopausal or postmenopausal status
          5. Symptoms of pelvic floor relaxation
      B. Male
          1. Prostate disorders
             a. Benign prostatic hypertrophy (BPH)
             b. Prostatitis
             c. Tumor
             d. Others
          2. Reproductive infections
             a. Sexually transmitted diseases
             b. Epididymo-orchitis
             c. Others
          3. Erectile function
          4. Ejaculatory function
  IV. Gastrointestinal system
      A. Frequency of bowel movements
      B. Typical stool consistency and caliber
      C. Patterns of bowel control
  V. General medical history
      A. Chronic conditions being treated
          a. Diabetes mellitus
          b. Hypertension
          c. Cancer
          d. Others
      B. Sensory disorders
          a. Loss of vision
          b. Hearing loss
          c. Others
  VI. Surgical history
  VII. Pharmacological assessment
      A. Prescription drugs
          a. Reason for prescription
          b. Duration of use
      B. Over-the-counter drugs
          a. Reason for use
          b. Duration of use

Source: Reprinted from Gray, M., Assessment of Patients with Urinary Incontinence, in *Urinary and Fecal Incontinence* by D. Doughty, p. 55, with permission of Mosby-Year Book, © 1991.

adults have not reported it to their physician (Burgio, Ives, Locher, Arena, & Kuller, 1994). Urinary incontinence is an embarrassing disorder, one with a strong social stigma associated with it. The older adult may be unable to discuss the problem objectively. During the first several decades of this century, the time when current older adults were growing up, it was not socially appropriate to discuss openly the problems of the genitourinary system. Also the older adult may express a sense of finality or resignation about the problem, stating that nothing can be done, or that previous health care providers had been unable to alleviate the disruption.

It is possible that an older adult may be inaccurate when reporting the amount of urine lost. Some researchers have reported that women after surgical treatment for urinary incontinence claimed vast improvement in the amount of urine lost. However, when urine loss was measured by the researchers, the amount of the loss was the same as before treatment (Warwick & Brown, 1979). Attitudes covering the spectrum from unconcern over a significant urine loss to dread of losing a few drops of urine exist in the older adult population. Objective measurement of actual urine loss (such as measuring the intake and output or preweighed pad tests) is necessary to make realistic plans for intervention.

Information about the personal consequences to the individual and what is used by the individual to manage the incontinence should be elicited. The Coping with Urinary Incontinence scale has been developed (Talbot, 1994). This is a 64-item self-reported scale that elicits information about an individual's effectiveness in coping with incontinence. See Chapter 6 about other measures of the psychological effects of urinary incontinence.

This information regarding the older adult's response to incontinence and the assessment process will provide important insights into the level of importance the problem and its solution is to the individual. It will also indicate the level of need for more education about incontinence and information about treatment options.

Throughout the assessment process, the health care provider must be patient and empathetic while providing accurate information and rationale for the procedures being performed. The health care provider must also be careful not to project a false sense of hope for a quick or complete cure. Assessment may be a time-consuming and, at times, a frustrating process. Emotional support and information to facilitate the older adult's means of coping are important components to the assessment process.

It is the obligation of the health care provider conducting the assessment to be sensitive to the affected person's feelings and level of discomfort. Providing an unhurried atmosphere that protects the individual's privacy, dignity, and comfort is essential to optimize the quality of the findings from the history and physical.

Caregiver and Living Environment Assessment

Whether the older adult is institutionalized or in the community, the attitude of the caregiver and/or family member must be assessed. If a fatalistic attitude such as "What can you expect at his/her age?" prevails, the nurse must address the issue when the care plan is being devised. Negative attitudes of the nursing staff or family members directed at the older adult have an impact on the older adult's functioning. The self-fulfilling prophecy of "I'll never be dry" can be inadvertently reinforced, thus a never-ending cycle of incontinence evolves.

As the history of the older adult is being taken, a description of the living environment should be obtained by direct observation and/or questioning. The distance from the bedroom to the bathroom, the older adult's level of mobility, and obstacles to access, such as stairs, dark hallways, and furniture should be addressed.

ASSESSMENT IN THE ACUTE CARE SETTING

Although nursing actions are intensive in the acute care setting and are focused on the primary reason for admission, assessment for urinary incontinence is possible. The nurse should establish the nature of the urinary incontinence: whether it is transient (symptom) or established (condition). Keeping a voiding record will provide important information about the pattern of incontinence. Obtaining a complete history using the form in Exhibit 4–2 will help to identify transient causes of incontinence. If the incontinence remains the same or worsens after treatment of the transient causes, further assessment may be required. This may occur in the acute care setting or may be performed on an outpatient basis after discharge.

VOIDING RECORD

Determination of the duration, pattern, and characteristics of incontinence is important and can be conducted at the same time as the history-taking phase. Using a voiding or bladder record is the simplest method to determine whether the incontinence is transient (symptom) or established (condition). The voiding record can help in characterizing the incontinence, in terms of the presence of dribbling, stress episodes, and urgency. However, the accuracy of the information is paramount. Every continent and incontinent void and its timing should be recorded for at least 3 days, or until a pattern emerges. There are many types of voiding records available. Exhibit 4–7 is one example. Voiding records that can fit easily into a shirt pocket or purse are preferable for active community-dwelling people. If a voiding record is being kept by the nursing staff, it may be kept at the bedside, covered to ensure privacy; each voiding should be recorded immediately after it occurs.

Exhibit 4–7 Voiding Record

Time	Amount Voided	Leakage	Amount of Fluid Consumed

Source: Reprinted from Gray, M., Assessment of Patients with Urinary Incontinence, in *Urinary and Fecal Incontinence* by D. Doughty, ed., p. 62, with permission of Mosby-Year Book, © 1991.

A computerized voiding record has been used to increase patient compliance and to facilitate analysis of the information. A portable unit is given to the individual with keys to be pressed in the event of an urge, an urge with leakage, leakage without an urge, a continent void, and ingestion of fluids (Rabin, McNett, & Badlani, 1993).

Cognitive Assessment

Prior to history taking, an assessment of the individual's cognitive status should be performed to determine the adequacy of short- and long-term memory, components necessary for the individual to provide a history. There are several quick, valid, and reliable cognitive screening tools. See Exhibit 4–8 for an example. If the individual has memory deficits, other sources of information will be needed, i.e., medical records, caregivers, family members, and other health care providers.

Exhibit 4–8 Instrument for Folstein "Mini-Mental State" Examination

Maximum Score	Score	Item
		Orientation
5	( )	What is the (year)(season)(date)(day)(month)?
5	( )	Where are we: (state)(county)(town)(hospital)(floor)?*
		Registration
3	( )	Name three objects: 1 second to say each. Then ask the patient all three after you have said them. Give 1 point for each correct answer. Then repeat them until he or she learns all three (for later checking).
		Attention and Calculation
5	( )	Serial 7s. Give 1 point for each correct. Stop after five answers. Alternatively spell *world* backwards.
		Recall
3	( )	Ask for the three objects repeated above. Give 1 point for each correct.
		Language
9	( )	Show patient a pencil and watch, and ask for their names. (2 points) Repeat the following: "No ifs, ands, or buts." (1 point) Follow a three-stage command: "Take a paper in your right hand, fold it in half, and put it on the floor." (3 points) Read and obey the following: "Close your eyes." (1 point) "Write a sentence." (1 point) "Copy a simple design." (1 point)

Total score

*The original wording of the item is listed here. In office practice, the terms *hospital* and *floor* might be replaced by such alternatives as *street* and *building*.

Source: Reprinted from Lachs, M. et. al., A Simple Procedure for General Screening for Functional Disability in Elderly Patients, *Annals of Internal Medicine*, Vol. 112, No. 9, p. 703, with permission of The American College of Physicians, © 1990.

Medications

The history should include information about both prescribed and over-the-counter drug use and other medical conditions. As noted in Chapter 3, many medications can contribute to incontinence. Anticholinergics, psychotropics, alpha-adrenergic agonists, and narcotic analgesics have a urinary retention effect. Alpha-adrenergic blockers relax the urethra.

Bowel and Urogenital Functioning

Information about bowel habits, occurrence of fecal incontinence, constipation, impaction, and bowel surgery should be obtained. History of previous urinary tract infections or urogenital complaints, such as dysuria, frequency, and urgency should also be elicited.

Because sphincter and pelvic floor competence play an important role in women's continence, women should be asked about their obstetrical history, especially the number of vaginal deliveries and the use of forceps during delivery. History of previous urogenital operations to repair prolapses or to correct incontinence are important as well. Postmenopausal women should be asked the date of their last menstrual period and their history of hormone replacement therapy. The smoking history should be elicited from women as well.

Smoking has been associated with incontinence (Bump & McClish, 1992). These authors postulated that the characteristic chronic and strong "smoker's cough" contributes to stress incontinence due to the severe pressure placed on the urethra and bladder neck during coughing. In addition, there may be long-term damage to the pelvic nerves from the downward stretching caused by the coughing. Tobacco may also have a direct adverse effect on collagen synthesis in the pelvic floor.

Men should be asked questions related to symptoms of benign prostatic hyperplasia. The American Urological Association has a symptoms inventory that consists of seven questions (Barry et al., 1992). Affirmative responses could indicate obstructive or irritative symptoms related to benign prostatic hyperplasia. See Exhibit 4–5 for the symptom index.

Physical Examination

A general examination of the person's overall physical condition should be undertaken (see Table 4–1). The presence of mobility impairments and manual dexterity problems could cause or exacerbate the severity of functional or urge incontinence. The individual's ability to transfer independently from bed to chair

Table 4–1 Procedure for Functional Assessment Screening in the Elderly

Target Area	Assessment Procedure	Abnormal Result	Suggested Intervention
Vision	Test each eye with Jaeger card while patient wears corrective lenses (if applicable).	Inability to read greater than 20/40	Refer to ophthalmologist.
Hearing	Whisper a short, easily answered question such as "What is your name?" in each ear while the examiner's face is out of direct view.	Inability to answer question	Examine auditory canals for cerumen and clean if necessary. Repeat test; if still abnormal in either ear, refer for audiometry and possible prosthesis.
Arm	Proximal: "Touch the back of your head with both hands." Distal: "Pick up the spoon."	Inability to do task	Examine the arm fully (muscle, joint, and nerve), paying attention to pain, weakness, limited range of motion. Consider referral for physical therapy.
Leg	Observe the patient after asking: "Rise from your chair, walk 10 feet, return, sit down."	Inability to walk or transfer out of chair	Do full neurological and musculoskeletal evaluation, paying attention to strength, pain, range of motion, balance, and traditional assessment of gait. Consider referral for physical therapy.
Urinary incontinence	Ask: "Do you ever lose your urine and get wet?"	Yes	Ascertain frequency and amount. Search for remediable causes including local irritations, polyuric states, and medications. Consider urologic referral.
Nutrition	Weigh the patient. Measure height.	Weight is below acceptable range for height	Do appropriate medical evaluation.

continues

Table 4-1 continued

Target Area	Assessment Procedure	Abnormal Result	Suggested Intervention
Mental status	Instruct: "I am going to name three objects (pencil, truck, book). I will ask you to repeat their names now and then again a few minutes from now." (See text discussion.)	Inability to recall all three objects after 1 minute	Administer Folstein mini-mental status examination. If score is <24, search for causes of cognitive impairment. Ascertain onset, duration, and fluctuation of overt symptoms. Review medications. Assess consciousness and affect. Do appropriate laboratory tests.
Depression	Ask: "Do you often feel sad or depressed?"	Yes	Administer Geriatric Depression Scale. If positive (normal score, 0 to 10), check for antihypertensive, psychotropic, or other pertinent medications. Consider appropriate pharmaceutical or psychiatric treatment.
ADL-IADL*	Ask: "Can you get out of bed yourself?", "Can you dress yourself?", "Can you make your own meals?", "Can you do your own shopping?"	No to any question	Corroborate responses with patient's appearance; question family members if accuracy is uncertain. Determine reasons for the inability (motivation compared with physical limitation). Institute appropriate medical, social, or environmental interventions.
Home environment	Ask: "Do you have trouble with stairs inside or outside of your home?"; ask about potential hazards inside the home with bathtubs, rugs, or lighting.	Yes	Evaluate home safety and institute appropriate countermeasures.

continues

Table 4–1 continued

Target Area	Assessment Procedure	Abnormal Result	Suggested Intervention
Social support	Ask: "Who would be able to help you in case of illness or emergency?"	...	List identified persons in the medical record. Become familiar with available resources for the elderly in the community.

*ADL-IADL = activities of daily living–instrumental activities of daily living.

Source: Reprinted from Lachs, M. et. al., A Simple Procedure for General Screening for Functional Disability in Elderly Patients, *Annals of Internal Medicine*, Vol. 112, No. 9, p. 700, with permission of The American College of Physicians, © 1990.

or from chair to commode is important to determine as well (Williams & Gaylord, 1990). The presence of sensory impairments such as visual or hearing impairments and neurological impairments, including abnormal reflexes, Parkinson's disease, and multiple sclerosis, should be assessed as well. Skin integrity, especially in the perineal area, should be assessed for excoriation and lesions. Pressure ulcers should be staged using a standardized method (Clinical Practice Guideline Panel, 1992b).

Physical assessment of the abdomen is an important part of the nursing assessment. This includes palpating for a distended bladder and/or bowel, observing the general abdominal muscle tone, and checking for the presence of scars from previous surgeries.

Physical Examination of Women

Visual examination of the urethra and vagina can reveal the presence of urethroceles, cystoceles, rectoceles, discharge, reddened thin epithelium lining, and atrophy of tissue. Manual examination can help determine the tone of the pelvic floor muscle and movement of the urethra and bladder neck in a downward, rotating direction when straining or coughing. The bulbocavernosus reflex should be elicited by gently touching the clitoris. Contraction of the rectal sphincter should result (McIntosh & Richardson, 1994). During the examination, discussion of personal hygiene habits with the woman should occur. The guidelines for client education are provided in Exhibit 4–9.

Physical Examination of Men

Visual examination of the glans should reveal a patent urethral meatus, and the foreskin, if present, should easily draw back (Kennedy & Steidle, 1991). A rectal exam is essential in assessing male incontinence. An enlarged prostate gland can obstruct the urethra sufficiently to cause overflow incontinence. Figure 4–2 provides a useful stepwise algorithm to evaluate incontinence in men. To determine whether urine is retained in the bladder after voiding, a postvoid residual (PVR) should be obtained. The bulbocavernosus reflex should be checked by gently squeezing the glans. Contraction of the rectal sphincter should result.

Urinalysis

The urinalysis is a valuable test in the assessment of incontinence. It will detect the presence of glycosuria, proteinuria, hematuria, pyuria, and bacteriuria (Fantl et al., 1996). Table 4–2 provides information about the interpretation of the results of a urinalysis performed on an older adult.

Exhibit 4-9 Guidelines for Good Personal Hygiene

1. Change to clean undergarments every day. If soiling occurs during the day, change after each episode.
2. Wear cotton or absorbent undergarments. Avoid tight-fitting panties and girdles. Panties with a wide leg may be more comfortable than panties with elastic legs.
3. Vinegar can be used in rinse water to help eliminate odor in undergarments. There are also commercial preparations available to help eliminate odor.
4. After voiding or bowel movements, wiping front to back with toilet tissue avoids contaminating the urethral and vaginal openings with pathogens or fecal material.
5. The perineal area should be cleansed at least once a day and after urine or stool incontinence. Warm water and limited use of a mild unscented soap helps to avoid drying out delicate perineal tissues. Rubbing with a washcloth or towel should be avoided. Patting the area dry with a towel prevents the irritation that rubbing can cause. It is essential for the perineal area to be kept clean and dry to prevent odor and skin excoriation.
6. Powder should be avoided in the perineal area. It can irritate perineal tissues and contribute to odor.
7. Purulent drainage, bleeding, foul-smelling exudate, and itching should be reported immediately to the health care provider.
8. Adequate oral intake (at least eight 8-ounce glasses a day) helps to keep the urine less concentrated and systemic tissues hydrated.
9. Avoid scented soap or perfumed toilet tissue to prevent irritation.
10. Avoid douching unless directed to do so by a health care provider.
11. Disposable pads and panty liners, if used, should be changed frequently and the skin assessed for irritation.

When bacteriuria is present and the person complains of the symptoms of a urinary tract infection, a specimen for culture and sensitivity should be obtained. Individuals should be given detailed instructions about cleansing the hands, the perineum, or glans to obtain a sterile specimen. Women should be instructed to hold the labia apart while obtaining the specimen. Care should be taken not to touch inside the specimen container or its lid.

Simple Urodynamic Evaluation

Assessment of Urine Flow

The assessment of urine flow is a noninvasive test in which urine flow is directly observed as the person voids. The person should have a comfortably full bladder, and the nurse should use a stopwatch to measure the length of time needed to complete voiding. This procedure can be embarrassing, causing the person difficulty in starting to void or emptying completely. Because delays in starting to

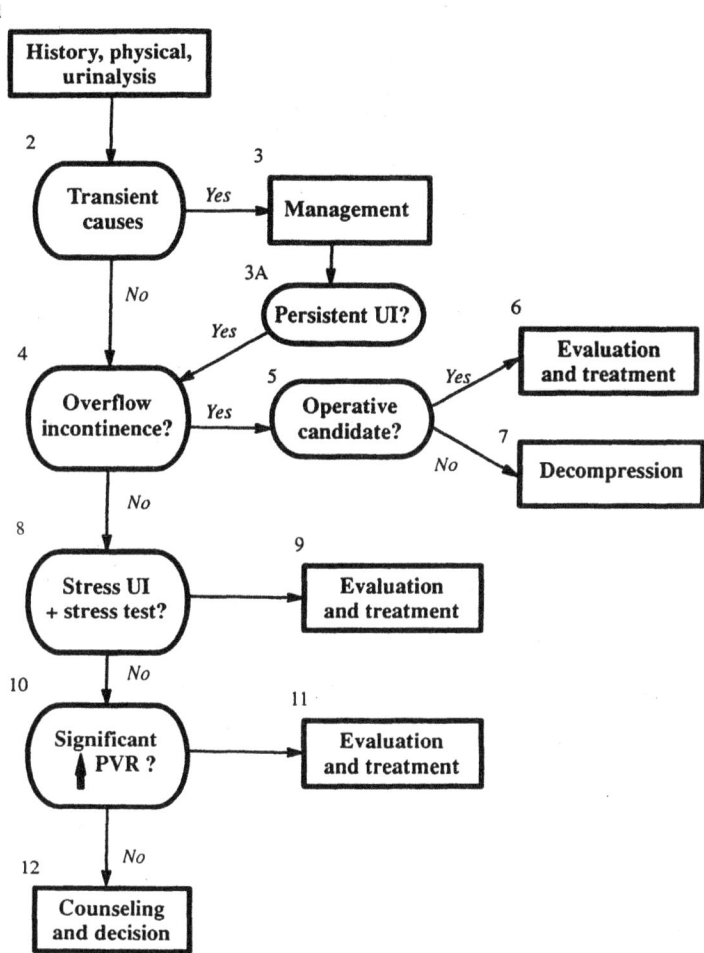

Figure 4–2 Algorithm for Assessment of Urinary Incontinence (UI) in Men. *Source:* Reprinted from Clinical Practice Guideline Panel, *Clinical Practice Guideline: Urinary Incontinence in Adults*, p. 82, Agency for Health Care Policy and Research, U.S. Department of Health and Human Services, Publication No. 92-0038, 1992.

void or prolonged time in emptying the bladder can be indicative of urinary retention, a technique whereby urine flow is measured in privacy is often preferred. In this case, the person is instructed to void into a uroflowmeter, and then is given the privacy to urinate. The uroflowmeter, a funnel-like device with electronic sensors that measure flow rate, can produce a graph of the individual's flow rate.

Table 4–2 Urinalysis: A Summary of Normal Values and Their Clinical Significance in the Elderly

Determination	Normal Value	Clinical Significance
Macroscopic Analysis		
Color	Pale yellow to dark amber	Very pale: diabetes insipidus, excess fluid intake, chronic renal disease, nervousness Very amber: dehydration Note: Medications may alter color
Appearance	Clear–slightly hazy	Cloudy, turbid: presence of bacteria, WBCs, or RBCs
Odor	Faintly aromatic	Fetid odor: bacterial infection Ammonia: urea breakdown by bacteria
Specific gravity	1.017–1.028	Decreased: overhydration; diabetes insipidus; diet (NA, PRO restriction) Elevated: ↓ fluid intake; fever; diabetes mellitus. ♦note: lower maximum value in the elderly
pH	4.5–8.0	>8.0: bacterial infection due to *Pseudomonas* or *Proteus*, chronic renal failure <4.5: metabolic/respiratory acidosis, starvation
Protein	Negative	Increased: renal disease, cardiac failure, febrile states, hematuria, amyloidosis
Glucose	Negative	Positive: uncontrolled diabetes mellitus; pituitary disorders; ↑ intracranial pressure. ♦Renal threshold for glucose rises after age 50, female > male.
Ketones	Negative	Positive: uncontrolled diabetes mellitus; prolonged vomiting; fasting
Blood	Negative	Positive: infection, renal calculus
Bilirubin	Negative	Positive: liver dysfunction
Nitrite	Negative	Positive: bacterial infection
Leukocyte esterase	Negative	Positive: pyuria
Microscopic Analysis		
RBCs	Rare per high power field	Increased: renal genitourinary disorders
WBCs	0–4 per high power field	Increased: bacterial infection ♦ not always a reliable indicator of infection in the elderly; if clinically asymptomatic is not significant

continues

Table 4-2 continued

Determination	Normal Value	Clinical Significance
Epithelial cells	0–3	Increased: probable perineal contamination
Casts	Rare per high power field	Increased: renal disease
Bacteria	<10^5 colonies/ml	Increased: bacterial infection ◆ significance is dependent upon specimen collection technique and specific gravity of sample

Source: Reprinted from Brazier, A. and Palmer, M., Collecting Clean-Caught Urine in the Nursing Home, *Geriatric Nursing,* Vol. 16, No. 5, pp. 217–224, Mosby-Year Book, 1995.

Uroflowmetry is useful in identifying problems in emptying, but it will not identify the location of the disruption (Wozniak-Petrofsky, 1995).

Pad Test

The pad test has been used to quantify urine loss (Victor, 1990; Wall, Wang, Robson, & Stanton, 1990; Rayome, 1995). Women are generally instructed to empty their bladder. They are then given a preweighed pad to wear for a specified period of time while performing activities that normally cause urine loss. The International Continence Society recommends 1 hour, although some researchers use a 2-hour time interval (Rayome, 1995). It should be noted that this test is highly sensitive in detecting incontinent women, but it may wrongly identify continent women as incontinent (Wall, Wang, Robson, & Stanton, 1990).

Postvoid Residual

To assess the adequacy of bladder emptying, the PVR is obtained after the person finishes voiding. The traditional method to determine how much urine remains in the bladder after voiding has been through straight catheterization. However, because of discomfort to the individual and the risk of introducing an infection or causing a urethral trauma, a portable ultrasound scanner can noninvasively and accurately detect the bladder contents (Newman & Smith, 1991). A PVR of ≤50 ml is considered adequate emptying. Several PVRs with volumes from 100 to 200 ml is considered inadequate (Fantl et al., 1996). Another indication of urinary retention is the PVR volume of 25% of the total bladder capacity (Rayome, 1995).

Simple Cystometrogram

A cystometrogram is a urodynamic procedure in which sterile fluid is introduced into the bladder via a catheter in a controlled manner. As the bladder is being filled, electronic readings are taken of the pressure in the bladder and the abdomen and are graphically displayed. By observing patterns of pressure, volume, detrusor contractions, patient sensations, and detrusor responses to provocative measures (coughing, straining), the neurological status of the bladder can be assessed. Thus, the cystometrogram serves as a very valuable tool for detecting the abnormal patterns of detrusor contraction characteristic of several types of incontinence.

Because the purpose of the cystometrogram is to evaluate the intravesical pressure-to-volume relationship during the filling/storage phase and the emptying phase, cystometry findings can provide graphic representation of the changes in pressure as the bladder fills. Figure 4–3 displays three patterns of filling: normal, urge, and overflow.

Normally as the bladder fills, there is little rise in pressure. At approximately 250 to 350 ml, the person usually reports the first indication of the need to void. Line *A* displays the rise of pressure as the bladder fills. A sudden rise in pressure, not represented in Figure 4–3, usually occurs between 400 and 600 ml, the functional capacity of the bladder (Byyny & Speroff, 1990). The tracing for an individual with a defect in the filling/storage phase due to an upper neuron lesion (above the sacral reflex center) is represented by line *B*. There are uninhibited bladder contractions at low bladder volume, and loss of urine at approximately 350 ml. The graphic representation of a defect in emptying due to a disruption in lower neuron functioning (sacral reflex center and lower) is displayed in line *C*. The bladder fills

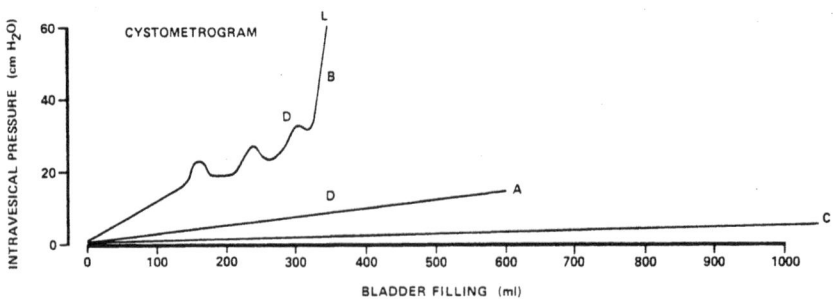

Figure 4–3 Representations of Various Cystometrograms. *A*, normal; *B*, uninhibited neurogenic or unstable bladder; *C*, a contractile bladder; *D*, first desire to void; *L*, leakage. *Source:* Reprinted from *Textbook of Geriatric Medicine and Gerontology*, 4th ed., by J. Brockelhurst, R. Tallis and H. Fillit, eds., p. 635, with permission of Churchill Livingstone, © 1992.

Assessment 75

to a tremendously large volume, over 1,000 ml, with no parallel rise in bladder pressure.

One of the simplest methods of cystometrics is to do an "eyeball" cystometrogram, which can be performed at the person's bedside or in a clinic setting (see Figure 4–4). Without electronic recording equipment, the clinician inserts a 12F or 16F catheter into an empty bladder; a large Toomey syringe is attached to the other end of the catheter, and a premeasured amount of sterile saline or sterile water is poured into the syringe. The bladder is filled by gravity. Early in the filling phase, fluid should flow easily into the bladder. The filling slows or fluid accumulates in the syringe as pressure rises. As with the more sophisticated cystometry discussed earlier, the person is instructed to report the first sensation of bladder fullness and

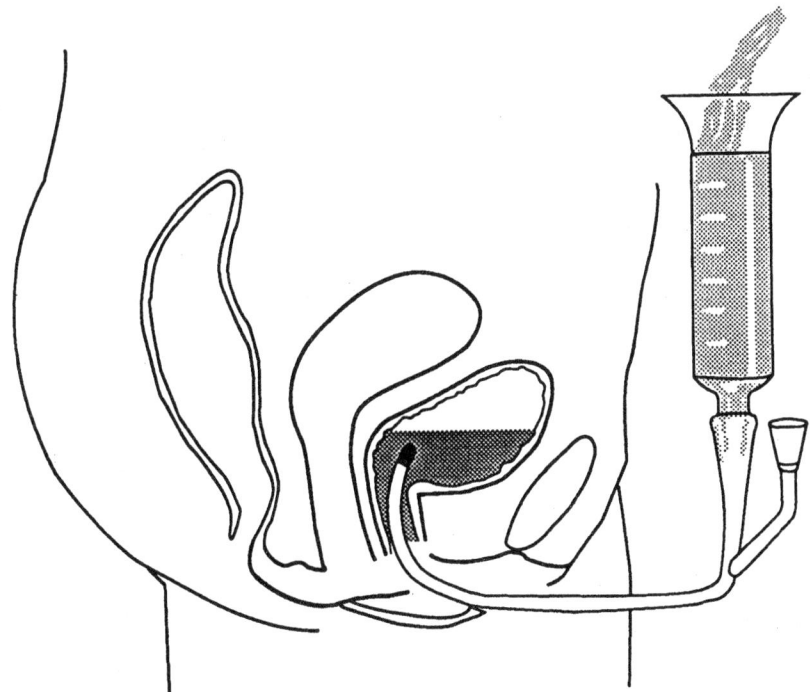

Figure 4–4 "Eyeball" Cystometrogram with Toomey Syringe and Catheter Can Be Performed in Clinic or Home Setting. *Source:* Reprinted from Rayome, R., Simple Urodynamic Techniques, *Journal of Wound, Ostomy and Continence Nursing*, Vol. 21, No. 1, p. 24, with permission of Mosby-Year Book, © 1995.

desire to void, as well as perform provocative measures to elicit uninhibited detrusor contractions or urinary leakage.

Invasive procedures always introduce the risk of infection and injury to the older adult. They should never be performed on a person without sterile urine. A person with a history of mitral valve prolapse or implants should be treated with prophylactic antibiotics prior to instrumentation of the urinary tract. An evaluation of the risks and benefits to the older adult must be carefully weighed before procedures are instituted.

CONCLUSION

Assessment of incontinence can be time consuming, expensive, and frustrating for the older adult. Many times there will be no "quick-fix." The older adult and health care team will expend a great deal of energy during the assessment of incontinence. Communication must be open among all health care professionals and with the older adult. The rationale for tests, explanations of terminology, and interpretations of test results are necessary ingredients of proper assessment. It is only through a comprehensive assessment of the causes of the urinary incontinence and consideration of the individual's readiness and preferences that decisions regarding treatment are made.

REFERENCES

Barry, M., Fowler, F., O'Leary, M., Bruskewitz, R., Holtgrewe, L., Mebust, W., Cockett, A., & the Measurement Committee of the American Urological Association. (1992). The American Urological Association symptom index for benign prostatic hyperplasia. *Journal of Urology, 148,* 1549–1557.

Brazier, A. (1994). Assessment of urinary incontinence in nursing homes: Level 2. *Nurse Practitioner Forum, 5*(3), 158–162.

Brazier, A., & Palmer, M. (1995). Collecting clean-caught urine in the nursing home: Obtaining the uncontaminated specimen. *Geriatric Nursing, 16,* 217–224.

Bump, R., & McClish, D. (1992). Cigarette smoking and urinary incontinence in women. *American Journal of Obstetrics and Gynecology, 167,* 1213–1218.

Burgio, K., Ives, D., Locher, J., Arena, V., & Kuller, L. (1994). Treatment seeking for urinary incontinence in older adults. *Journal of the American Geriatrics Society, 42,* 208–212.

Byyny, R., & Speroff, L. (Eds.). (1990). The urinary tract and pelvic floor. In *A clinical guide for the care of older women.* Baltimore: Williams & Wilkins.

Callahan, C., Hui, S., Nienaber, N., Musick, B., & Tierney, W. (1994). Longitudinal study of depression and health services use among elderly primary care patients. *Journal of the American Geriatrics Society, 42,* 833–838.

Clinical Practice Guideline Panel. (1992a). *Clinical practice guideline: Urinary incontinence in adults* (AHCPR Pub. No. 92-0038). Rockville, MD: Agency for Health Care Policy and Research, Public Health Service, U.S. Department of Health and Human Services.

Clinical Practice Guideline Panel. (1992b). *Clinical practice guideline: Pressure ulcers in adults: Prediction and prevention* (AHCPR Pub. No. 92-0047). Rockville, MD: Agency for Health Care Policy and Research, Public Health Service, U.S. Department of Health and Human Services.

Fantl, J.A., Newman, D.K., & Colling, J. et al. (1996). Urinary incontinence in adults: Acute and chronic management. *Clinical practice guideline no. 2, 1996 update.* (AHCPR Pub. No. 96-0692). Rockville, MD: Agency for Health Care Policy and Research, Public Health Service, U.S. Department of Health and Human Services.

Fox, R. (1988). Atypical presentation of geriatric infections. *Geriatrics, 43,* 58–68.

Kane, R., Ouslander, J., & Abrass, I. (1994). Incontinence. In *Essentials of clinical geriatrics* (3rd ed.). New York: McGraw-Hill.

Kennedy, K., & Steidle, C. (1991, July/August). Achieving a state of urinary continence for residents of nursing facilities. *Ostomy/wound management, 35,* 72–77.

Kinney, A., Blount, M., & Dowell, M. (1980). Urethral catheterization. *Geriatric Nursing, 1,* 258–263.

Koenig, H., & Blazer, D. (1991). Mood disorders and suicide. In J. Birren, R. Sloane, & G. Cohen (Eds.), *Handbook of mental health and aging* (2nd ed.). New York: Academic Press.

McGeer, A., Campbell, B., Emori, T., Hierhoizer, W., Jackson, M., Nicolle, L. et al. (1991). Definitions of infections for long-term care facilities. *American Journal of Infection Control, 19,* 1–7.

McIntosh, L., & Richardson, D. (1994). 30-Minute evaluation of incontinence in the older woman. *Geriatrics, 42,* 35–44.

Newman, D., & Smith, D. (1991). A portable bladder scanner. *Nurse Practitioner Forum, 2,* 243–245.

Nicolle, L. (1993). Urinary tract infections in long-term care facilities. *Infection Control and Hospital Epidemiology, 14,* 220–225.

Ouslander, J., Morishita, L., Blaustein, J., Orzeck, S., Dunn, S., & Sayre, J. (1987). Clinical, functional, and psychological characteristics of an incontinent nursing home population. *Journal of Gerontology, 42,* 631–637.

Ouslander, J., Schapira, M., & Schnelle, J. (1995). Urine specimen collection from incontinent female nursing home residents. *Journal of the American Geriatrics Society, 43,* 279–281.

Ouslander, J., Simmons, S., Tuico, E., Nigam, J., Fingold, S., Bates-Jensen, B., & Schnelle, J. (1994). Use of a portable ultrasound device to measure post-void residual volume among incontinent nursing home residents. *Journal of the American Geriatrics Society, 42,* 1189–1192.

Palmer, M. (1994). Level 1: Basic assessment and management of urinary incontinence in nursing homes. *Nurse Practitioner Forum, 5*(3), 152–157.

Rabin, J., McNett, J., & Badlani, G. (1993). Computerized voiding diary. *Neurology and Urodynamics, 12,* 541–554.

Radloff, L. (1977). The CES-D Scale: A self-report depression scale for research in the general population. *Applied Psychological Measurement, 1,* 385–401.

Rayome, R. (1995). Simple urodynamic techniques. *Journal of Wound, Ostomy and Continence Nursing, 22,* 17–26.

Schultz, B., & Gambert, S. (1991). Influence of chronic disease on the presentation of urinary tract infections in the institutionalized elderly. *Age, 14*, 79–81.

Talbot, L. (1994). Coping with urinary incontinence: Development and testing of a scale. *Nursing Diagnosis, 5*(3), 127–132.

Varney, H. (1987). *Nurse midwifery* (2nd ed.). Cambridge, MA: Blackwell-Scientific.

Victor, A. (1990). Pad weighing test—a simple method to quantitate urinary incontinence. *Annals of Medicine, 22*, 443–447.

Wall, L., Wang, K., Robson, I., & Stanton, S. (1990). The pyridium pad test for diagnosing urinary incontinence. *Journal of Reproductive Medicine, 35*, 682–684.

Warwick, R., & Brown, A. (1979). A urodynamic evaluation of urinary incontinence in the female and its treatment. *Symposium in Clinical Urodynamics, 6*, 203–216.

Williams, M., & Gaylord, S. (1990). Role of functional assessment in the evaluation of urinary incontinence. *Journal of the American Geriatrics Society, 38*, 296–299.

Wozniak-Petrofsky, J. (1995). Basic elements of urodynamic evaluation in urinary incontinence. *Urologic Nursing, 14*(3), 125–129.

Wyman, J. (1988). Nursing assessment of the incontinent geriatric outpatient population. *Nursing Clinics of North America, 23*, 169–187.

CHAPTER

5

Treatment

Effective treatment for urinary incontinence is possible. However, incontinence must be detected by a health care provider, or the older adult must seek treatment. Unfortunately, some incontinent older adults do not seek treatment, believing that the incontinence is an inevitable part of aging (Burgio, Ives, Locher, Arena, & Kuller, 1994). Public education about the causes of incontinence and the multiple treatment options available for incontinence is an essential component of effective continence promotion programs.

This chapter discusses behavioral, pharmacological, and surgical treatment options available for the most common causes of urinary incontinence in older adults. Treatment for incontinence in the long-term care, the home care, and the acute settings is also briefly discussed. A detailed presentation of surgical options is beyond the scope of this book. The reader is referred to current urological texts for the various surgical procedures used to correct anatomical defects. Table 5–1 provides the reader with a quick overview of the types, causes, assessment, and treatments of urinary incontinence. Absorbent products, equipment, and other devices are discussed in Chapter 8.

GENERAL GUIDELINES

Treatment for urinary incontinence follows a thorough assessment of the causes of and factors related to the incontinence. A basic understanding of the pathophysiology of incontinence is needed by all individuals involved in the treatment and care plan. The affected older adult should be included in the decision-making process. Besides considering the older adult's lifestyle and preferences for treatment, other factors should be weighed before treatment is implemented. These include the risks, benefits, and outcomes of different treatment options. The

Table 5-1 Overview of the Causes, Assessment, and Treatment of Urinary Incontinence (UI)

Type of UI	Cause	Assessment	Treatment
		Urological/Gynecological	
Overflow	Failure to empty: Prostatic hyperplasia	History of hesitancy, dribbling, and less forceful stream, sensation of incomplete emptying Detailed medical history Digital rectal exam Focused neurological exam Prostate-specific antigen test Voiding record Urinalysis, urine culture and sensitivity Serum creatinine	Resection of prostate Balloon dilation Alpha-blockers Avoidance of anticholinergic drugs Intermittent catheterization Suprapubic catheterization
Stress	Failure to store: Weak pelvic musculature, organ prolapse, urethral hypermobility, intrinsic sphincter deficiency	History of vaginal deliveries History of sensation of pelvic fullness, urinary leakage with cough or sneeze Evidence of urine loss with provocation Evidence of urethral hypermobility Pelvic exam Pad test Pelvic muscle strength Urinalysis Urine culture and sensitivity	Pelvic floor training Biofeedback Hormone replacement therapy Weight loss, if obese Surgical intervention Electrical stimulation Medication Management of chronic respiratory diseases Periurethral bulking injections

continues

Table 5-1 continued

Type of UI	Cause	Assessment	Treatment
Urge	Failure to store: Urinary tract infection Vaginitis Bladder stones Bladder tumors	History of burning, dysuria, frequency, urgency, or hematuria Urinalysis Urine culture and sensitivity Assess perineal hygiene Pelvic exam, smear of vaginal discharge Cystometrogram	Antimicrobial medication Antiseptic medications Topical estrogen therapy Hygiene education Increased oral fluids Removal of bladder stones Resection of tumors
		Neurological	
Urge	Failure to store: Cortical, subcortical, and suprasacral lesions Cerebrovascular accident, dementia Parkinson's disease Multiple sclerosis	Assess mental status Assess ability to delay voiding History of nocturia, frequency, inability to delay voiding, urgency Evidence of large amount of urine loss with each episode Neurological exam Voiding record Cystogram with evidence of uninhibited bladder contractions with or without impaired emptying Defects in inhibition Decreased bladder capacity May exhibit lack of synchronization between detrusor contraction and sphincter function	Scheduled toileting Prompted voiding Bladder training Improve mobility Bowel training Biofeedback Medication Collection devices, urinals Management of fluid intake Intermittent catheterization

continues

Treatment 81

Table 5-1 continued

Type of UI	Cause	Assessment	Treatment
Urge	Failure to store: Spinal cord transection due to infection, neoplasm, or trauma	Evidence of unstable detrusor with decreased capacity Inhibition of micturition absent, no sensation of fullness, no volitional control	Anticholinergic medication Intermittent catheterization
Overflow	Failure to empty: Diabetes mellitus Tabes dorsalis Sacral spinal cord lesion	History of constipation Voiding record Large postvoid residual Cystogram No sensation of fullness, no volitional control Urinalysis Urine culture Focused neurological examination	Treatment of acute underlying conditions Credé maneuver Scheduled toileting Medications Intermittent catheterization
		Internal Environment	
Functional	Effects of medications: diuretics, hypnotics, alcohol, narcotics, decongestants, cold and allergy medications	History of drug/alcohol use Medication history, including time of administration Voiding record Assess fluid intake and output Assess sleep patterns Assess postvoid residual Assess access to toilet	Rescheduled medication and fast-acting diuretics earlier in the day Decreased use of hypnotics Decreased use of alcohol Avoidance of anticholinergic drugs Easy access to toilet High-fiber diet, exercise, and adequate hydration

continues

Table 5-1 continued

Type of UI	Cause	Assessment	Treatment
Functional	Manual dexterity/mobility	History of chronic disease, e.g., arthritis Assess functional status Assess living environment Assess ability to use toilet	Treatment of underlying disease Easy-to-remove clothing Convenient toilet facilities Urinals and commodes Proper prosthetic devices: canes, walkers, shoes Pain management Prompted voiding Scheduled toileting Physical therapy
Transient	Delirium	Assess for physiological alterations Assess for sleep deprivation Assess for fecal impaction Assess mental status Measure fluid intake and output Assess for infection Assess for an overstimulating environment	Treatment of underlying cause Checking and changing until sensorium clears Scheduled toileting Promotion of self-esteem Urinals, commodes, collection devices
Functional	Sensory deficits	Screening of hearing and vision Neurological function	Eyeglasses, hearing aids, and proper lighting Easy-to-read signs Low ambient sounds Prompted voiding Scheduled toileting Urinals and commodes Habit training

continues

Table 5-1 continued

Type of UI	Cause	Assessment	Treatment
Transient	Fecal impaction	History of constipation Bowel habits Defecation pattern Laxative abuse	High-fiber diet, exercise, and adequate hydration Regular evacuation
Transient	Medical conditions: Uncontrolled diabetes mellitus	Onset of diabetes mellitus Monitor blood glucose Urinalysis Urine culture Fluid intake and output Voiding record Assess peripheral sensation	Diabetes mellitus management Scheduled toileting Personal hygiene Intermittent catheterization if chronic
		External Environment	
Functional	Inadequate toilet facilities Bulky clothing	Check distance to toilet Assess environment for toilet accessibility Assess ability to disrobe for toileting Maintain voiding record	Proper commode height Toilet seat riser arm rails Velcro fasteners Loose-fitting clothing Privacy Easy access to toilet Provision of commode, urinals, external collection devices Labeled toilet locations Prompted voiding Scheduled toileting Habit training

continues

Table 5-1 continued

Type of UI	Cause	Assessment	Treatment
Functional	Use of physical restraints	Assess need and benefits of restraints Assess access to toilet facilities	Removal of restraints Close supervision if medical condition requires restraints Scheduled toileting Easy access to toilet substitutes Out-of-bed toileting as soon as condition permits

first treatment choice should be the least invasive and pose the least risk to the patient (Fantl, Newman, & Colling et al., 1996).

The current general health status and previous medical history of the older adult are important factors in determining whether specific surgical procedures and pharmacological agents are appropriate and can be tolerated. Assessment of the cognitive status is essential before initiating options involving participation and cooperation of the older adult. These options include administering medications, following a voiding schedule, using or changing external devices, keeping a voiding record, and performing specific exercises. Some treatment options, such as behavioral therapies that require some mobility to gain access to the toilet and using and changing external collection devices, are inappropriate for older adults with limited mobility and impaired manual dexterity.

The motivational level of the individual should be assessed. Behavioral treatments, such as pelvic muscle exercises, may take several weeks of consistent adherence before treatment effects are observed. Helping the incontinent older adult allay anxiety about incontinence is an important part of any treatment option. Feelings of hopelessness, frustration, and anxiousness can compound the intensity of the problem and confound treatment. Devising means of coping, such as ventilating concerns and feelings to a caring listener, physical exercising, and participating in pleasurable activities are all appropriate for the older adult. Before treatment begins, the goals of the older adult must be understood. Various goals may be held, from complete continence to reducing the number of incontinent episodes (Sale & Wyman, 1994).

One of the most important components of any treatment is the promotion of the individual's self-esteem and maintenance of a high level of motivation in the older adult. Having attractive clothing to wear and friendly, warm surroundings promotes not only self-esteem but continent behavior by the older adult. Clean and private toilet facilities also act as a cue to the incontinent older adult that continence is a desirable state. Realistic goal setting in terms of the individual's level of functioning will prevent overoptimistic anticipation and inflated expectations of outcome for the treatment.

In the course of assessment and treatment of incontinence, health care providers may find some individuals who are relatively unconcerned by their incontinence and have poor personal hygiene habits. It can be difficult to effect changes of behavior in these individuals to promote continence. The staff must approach these individuals with empathy, a nonjudgmental attitude, and respect for the free will of the individual. Using this approach, treatment consists of counseling sessions with the individual in which expectations of the caregiver and older adult are clearly understood. An agreement, or contract, is made by both parties in which the individual gains or retains control over certain aspects of his or her lifestyle while modifying behaviors to meet standards the caregiver sets. While this procedure sounds fairly straightforward, it can be a time-consuming and, at times, a frustrating process. The caregivers must come to care planning meetings with realistic expectations and a willingness to modify them. The attitude that "he/she is going to do this or else" sets the stage for failure. When communications break down, there is alienation of the individual and few alternatives are left. The temptation to control another's behavior absolutely must be avoided by the caregivers. The older adult must be afforded the opportunity to change or modify his or her own behavior. This can be done through joint decision making and negotiation. Realistic and mutual goals set through the negotiation process, genuine interest and empathy by caregivers, and reinforcement with actions or objects of value to the individual are effective techniques in the treatment of urinary incontinence.

BEHAVIORAL TREATMENT

Pelvic Floor Training

Pelvic floor training is used to treat stress incontinence secondary to pelvic floor incompetence with or without prolapse. The International Continence Society (ICS) Committee on Standardisation of Terminology (1992) defined pelvic floor training as "repetitive selective volitional contractions and relaxations of specific pelvic floor muscles" (p. 8). In order to correctly perform pelvic muscle training, the individual must be able to differentiate between the target muscle contraction and unwanted contractions of nearby or adjacent muscle groups. The most commonly known pelvic muscle training method is the Kegel exercises, or pelvic muscle exercises.

In the late 1940s Kegel developed a perineometer, a device placed in the vagina that acted as passive resistance to contractions of the pelvic floor, to help postpartum women strengthen their pelvic muscles (Wells, 1990). The goal of pelvic muscle exercise is to increase the strength of the pubococcygeus portion of the levator ani to effect efficient urethral closure during periods of sudden and sharp intravesical pressure, e.g., during coughing, straining, etc. (Miller, Kasper, & Sampselle, 1994). Expected outcomes of pelvic muscle exercise are increased strength and size of the pubococcygeus; increased duration of muscle contraction with corresponding increase in urethral pressure; decrease of urine loss during urodynamic testing involving provocative maneuvers; increase in the ability to stop urine flow once it is initiated; self-report of decrease in urine loss, increase in self-esteem, and enhanced quality of life; and decrease in reliance on pads, panty liners, or other absorbent products.

Because pelvic muscle exercise is a learned technique of target muscle contraction and relaxation, women must be motivated to learn the exercises and practice them daily. Initially, the woman must be able to identify correctly the target muscles and master the ability to perform short flicks of contraction as well as sustain contractions. There are two muscle layers being exercised when the different types of contraction take place. Type II muscle fibers produce fast and strong contractions, while type I fibers produce sustained contractions, less intense than those produced by type II fibers. After the woman has mastered contraction of the correct muscles, strength training of these muscles begins; increasing the duration of the contraction becomes the next phase of the exercise regimen. Once the woman's goal of strength or continence is attained, a reduced level of exercise must continue to maintain the strength of the muscles (Miller et al., 1994).

Therefore, compliance with the exercise program is critical to its success. It is recommended that the woman begin with 10 exercises daily, increasing by 10 exercises each week until at least 40 to 60 exercises are performed daily (Newman & Smith, 1992). Each contraction should be sustained for 10 seconds. See Exhibit 5–1 for an example of instructions for pelvic muscle exercise. Sometimes topical estrogen cream is prescribed in conjunction with pelvic muscle exercise to relieve symptoms of atrophic vaginitis and to replenish vaginal and urethral tissue.

In an attempt to alleviate pressure on the bladder and pelvic floor, overweight and obese women should receive instruction about nutrition, weight management, and physical exercise. Constricting undergarments such as tight girdles should be avoided as well.

Pelvic muscle exercise has been used to treat urge incontinence as well. It is postulated that these exercises cause neuromuscular changes resulting in a decrease of autocontractility of the detrusor, thus allaying urge incontinence (Flynn, Cell, & Luisi, 1994).

Pelvic muscle exercise has been combined with biofeedback to improve pelvic floor tone and to reduce uninhibited bladder contractions. Biofeedback is defined as "a technique by which information about a normally unconscious physiological process is presented to the patient and the therapist as a visual, auditory, or tactile signal. The signal is derived from a measurable physiological parameter which is subsequently used in an educational process to accomplish a specific therapeutic result" (ICS Committee, 1992, p. 100).

Pelvic muscle activity can be measured as changes in pressure (manometry) and changes in electrical activity (electromyography). Changes in pressure during muscle contraction can be determined during an exercise with biofeedback session by insertion of a probe into the vagina or into the rectum. To determine electrical activity in pelvic floor and abdominal muscles, surface electrodes are placed around the anus and on the abdomen below the umbilicus (Smith & Newman, 1994). Visual displays of changes in pressure during the training session allow the biofeedback therapist to provide immediate feedback to the older adult regarding

Exhibit 5–1 Instructions for Pelvic Muscle Exercises

PELVIC MUSCLE (KEGEL) EXERCISES

- HOW TO FIND THE PELVIC MUSCLE

  Imagine you are at a party and the rich food you have just eaten causes you to have gas or to pass "wind." The muscle that you use to hold back gas is the pelvic muscle. Some people find this muscle by trying to stop their stream of urine. Another way to find the muscle is by pulling your rectum, vagina, or urethra up inside your body.

- EXERCISING THE MUSCLE

  Begin by emptying your bladder. Then try to relax completely. Tighten your pelvic muscle and hold for a count of 10 or for 10 seconds, then relax the muscle completely for a count of 10 or for 10 seconds. You should feel a lifting sensation in the area around the vagina or a pulling in your rectum.

- WHEN TO EXERCISE

  Do your exercise three times a day, 10 exercises in the morning, 10 in the afternoon, and 15 at night. Or you can exercise for 10 minutes, three times a day. You can use a kitchen timer to time yourself.

- WHAT IF I CANNOT SQUEEZE FOR 10 SECONDS?

  At first you may not be able to squeeze for a count of 10, so squeeze for a count of 5 and relax for 5. In time, increase squeezing to 10 seconds. If the muscle starts to tire after six or eight exercises, stop and go back to exercising later.

- WHERE TO PRACTICE THESE EXERCISES

  These exercises can be practiced anywhere and anytime. Most people like to exercise lying on their bed or sitting in a chair. Women can even do these exercises during sexual intercourse. Tighten pelvic muscles to grip your partner's penis and then relax. Your partner should be able to feel an increase in pressure. If you have a "Bladder Exercise" tape, listen to it twice a day and follow the instructions.

- COMMON MISTAKES

  Never use your stomach, legs, or buttocks muscles. Put your hand on your stomach when you squeeze your pelvic muscle. If you feel your stomach move, then you are also using these muscles. Your legs and buttocks muscles should not move.

- CAN THESE EXERCISES HURT ME?

  NO! These exercises cannot harm you in any way. You should find them relaxing and easy. If you get back pain or stomach pain after you exercise, then you are probably trying too hard and using stomach muscles. If you experience headaches, then you are also tensing your chest muscles and probably holding your breath.

- WHEN WILL I NOTICE A CHANGE?

  After 4 to 6 weeks of consistent daily exercise, you will begin to notice less urinary leakage and after 3 months you will see an even bigger difference. Make these exercises part of your lifestyle. Tighten the muscle when you walk, before you cough, as you stand up, and on the way to the bathroom.

Source: Copyright © 1994, Access to Continence Care & Treatment, Inc., Saint Davids, Pennsylvania.

efficient contractions of the appropriate muscles. Contraction of the abdominal muscles while contracting the pelvic floor muscle is discouraged because these contractions only increase intra-abdominal pressure (Tries, 1990).

The goal of pelvic muscle exercise with biofeedback for treatment of stress incontinence is to teach the individual to contract periurethral muscles while simultaneously decreasing abdominal contraction. An adjunct device, vaginal weights, may sometimes be used as a part of pelvic muscle exercise. Vaginal weights are tampon-sized and -shaped devices with a nylon tether at the distal end to facilitate removal. They generally come in sets of five, in a series of graduated weights (Newman & Smith, 1992). Vaginal weights have been used to aid women in learning to identify correctly which muscles to contract as they begin a pelvic muscle program (Miller et al., 1994) or as a separate exercise program (Newman & Smith, 1992). To avoid infections when vaginal weights are used, weights should never be shared and women must be instructed to insert a vaginal weight with clean hands and to cleanse and dry the weights thoroughly after each use.

When pelvic muscle exercise with biofeedback is used to treat urge incontinence, changes in detrusor pressure and/or muscle electrical activity can be visually displayed as the bladder is filled with sterile water or sterile saline. The individual, with the assistance of the biofeedback therapist, can identify uninhibited contractions. The individual is taught abdominal muscle relaxation techniques to suppress these contractions while contracting the pelvic floor muscle to prevent urine loss during an uninhibited contraction (Burgio & Engel, 1990).

Biofeedback techniques vary, but the underlying principle is the same. The individual watches a graphic display on a video monitor of their own bladder filling. The individual's physiologic response to contract the periurethral muscles and/or to counteract an uninhibited contraction is also recorded, providing feedback regarding the effectiveness of the attempts at control. After a series of sessions, the individual learns which efforts are most effective in contracting the pelvic muscle or counteracting contractions of the detrusor.

Men with urge incontinence or stress incontinence due to sphincter incompetence after surgical removal of the prostate can benefit from pelvic muscle exercise with or without biofeedback.

Individuals must be prepared for the prolonged nature of the treatment, be willing to comply with the exercise schedule, and be comfortable with the invasive nature of the pelvic muscle exercise and biofeedback program (Housten, 1993). During pelvic muscle exercise treatment for incontinence, the use of sanitary pads and continence pads and briefs should be discouraged. The use of pads and briefs blunt the sensation of wetness (Coxe, 1994), and there may be a psychological dependency on these products that could counter the therapeutic effects of the pelvic muscle exercise treatment.

Behavioral Modification

There are several behavioral therapies designed to modify an incontinent older adult's behavior. The International Continence Society defined behavioral modification as comprising "analysis and alteration of the relationship between the patient's symptoms and his/her environment for the treatment of maladaptive voiding patterns" (ICS Committee, 1992, p. 101). Before any behavioral therapy is implemented, a thorough assessment of the individual's incontinence, general health, and environment must be performed. Factors that occur prior to an incontinent episode must be assessed as well. These include an individual's ability to discern bladder fullness and the ability to communicate the need to use the toilet, as well as the physical ability to gain access to the toilet. There are strong antecedent cues to empty the bladder, such as the sensation of bladder fullness, the sight of a toilet, and sitting on an open seat while not wearing underwear (Palmer, 1990). Caregivers must be keenly aware of these and other antecedent verbal and nonverbal factors in the environment that promote or hinder continence.

Besides assessing the antecedent factors, the consequences of incontinent behavior must be considered. If an incontinent older adult receives social and physical contact only during changing and cleaning after an incontinent episode, then the caregiver may be unconsciously reinforcing that behavior.

The goal of each behavioral modification therapy must be weighed and matched as closely as possible to the individual's goals and capabilities. For example, an individual unable to delay voiding because of underlying pathology or dementia is not an appropriate candidate for interventions that require some potential for voluntary control over micturition.

The behavioral modification therapies most frequently used are bladder training, prompted voiding, scheduled toileting, and habit training. These interventions can be used alone or in conjunction with other therapies, e.g., pharmacological interventions. With the exception of prompted voiding, these interventions may be totally self-managed by the individual or initiated by the staff.

Bladder Training

Bladder training, a behavioral modification treatment for urge incontinence, has also been called bladder retraining or bladder drill. The purpose of bladder training is to restore a normal pattern of voiding and normal bladder function (Palmer & McCormick, 1991). Expected outcomes of bladder training are a decrease in number of wet episodes, a decrease in the amount of urine lost, a decrease in the number of voidings, an increase in bladder capacity, and an increase in quality of life. The purpose of bladder training is to inhibit involuntary detrusor contractions (Fantl et al., 1991).

The individual is given instruction about normal micturition with emphasis on central or cortical control and the assigned fixed voiding schedule. Initially the person is instructed to void at fixed intervals, usually every 30 to 60 minutes, regardless of whether the urge to void is present. If an urge to void occurs before the next scheduled time to void, the person is instructed to suppress this urge by using relaxation or distracting activities. The individual keeps a voiding record and records continent and incontinent voidings and their timing. Each week the time interval is increased by 30 minutes until a normal voiding pattern is established, e.g., every 3 to 4 hours. Anticholinergic medications can be used in conjunction with bladder training of unstable bladders. Tricyclic antidepressants used to alleviate symptoms of anxiety and depression (common in older adults) also have the effect of increasing urinary retention. This side effect can be of benefit to some individuals with urge incontinence.

It is postulated that bladder training works through various mechanisms, one of which is that the increase in cerebral inhibition of contraction also improves sphincter function. Another postulated mechanism is that the changes in toileting lead to more acute awareness of behavior and influences changes in behavior regarding toileting (Fantl et al., 1991). Cognitively impaired older adults who are unable to understand and retain instructions about bladder training or who are unable to inhibit voiding may not be appropriate for this intervention.

Scheduled Toileting

Scheduled toileting is used to treat urge and functional incontinence. The individual is offered the use of a toilet, urinal, or bedpan every 2 to 4 hours. The purpose of scheduled toileting, a fixed schedule for emptying the bladder, is to avoid incontinent episodes. There are no attempts to regain a normal voiding pattern, and the schedule for toileting is not based on the sensation of bladder fullness. Expected outcomes for scheduled toileting include a decrease in number of wet episodes, a decrease in laundry costs and use of absorbent products, an improved quality of life, and an increase in social activities.

Habit Training

Habit training involves using a schedule for toileting that is based on the individual's voiding pattern for the entire day, not just waking hours. Colling, Ouslander, Hadley, Eisch, and Campbell (1992) described patterned urge-response toileting (PURT), a method of discerning an individual's voiding pattern and providing toileting assistance based on this pattern.

Before habit training begins, the nursing staff observes the individual's voiding pattern using a bladder record or bladder log for 3 days. For some individuals, voiding times are similar from one day to another, especially for individuals who ingest fluids, take meals, and retire at a routine time every day (Colling et al., 1992).

The nursing staff offers access to the toilet or toilet substitute at times that best approximate the times of voiding noted during the observation phase of the intervention. Habit training is an appropriate intervention for cognitively impaired individuals with functional, urge, or a combination of stress and urge incontinence who can cooperate with toileting. Expected outcomes for habit training are decreased frequency of incontinent episodes, increased comfort, and increased quality of life by the individual. Environmental modifications, as discussed in Chapter 8, should be implemented as well to provide easy access to the toilet.

Prompted Voiding

Prompted voiding is an effective behavioral modification for the treatment of urge and functional incontinence in individuals who have few incontinent episodes, are able to cooperate with toileting, are able to respond to prompts to use the toilet, and are able to inhibit urination. The purpose of prompted voiding is to heighten the individual's awareness of the need to void, increase interactions between the caregiver and the individual, prevent wet episodes, and ensure caregiver adherence to the prompted voiding schedule through a method of staff performance feedback.

Prompted voiding employs a toileting schedule, verbal feedback, and reinforcement. Expected outcomes include a decrease in wet episodes, an increase in dryness, an increase in quality of life, an increase in access to the toilet, an increase in awareness of the need to void, and high caregiver adherence to the schedule. Prompted voiding is a two-pronged approach to increasing dryness and reducing wet episodes. One prong of the intervention is directed toward the incontinent older adult; the other is focused on the caregiver. On a fixed or variable schedule the older adult is approached by the caregiver and the following five activities occur:

1. The caregiver approaches at the specified time and asks the individual whether he or she is wet or dry.
2. The caregiver physically checks the individual for accuracy of the response.
3. The caregiver provides verbal feedback about the accuracy of the answer.

4. The caregiver offers the older adult assistance to the toilet or toilet substitute.
5. After toileting and repositioning the older adult, the caregiver reminds the older adult about the next scheduled check and encourages the older adult to call for help with toileting if needed.

If assistance is refused, a person should never be forced to use the toilet (Palmer, Bennett, Marks, McCormick, & Engel, 1994). In order for prompted voiding to be effective, the caregiver must be scrupulous in offering toileting assistance as scheduled. Therefore, in an institutional setting, the second prong of the prompted voiding approach, staff feedback mechanisms, is employed.

Schnelle (1991) developed a prompted voiding intervention with a quality control method for long-term care facilities in which the incontinent person's average number and standard deviation of incontinent episodes are calculated at the beginning of the intervention. This information is used as a quality indicator for the administrators of the facility and for the staff to evaluate the effectiveness of the intervention.

Another method of prompted voiding employs the Behavioral Supervision Model (Burgio, 1994). This method includes defined responsibilities of staff members for the prompted voiding intervention, individualized verbal feedback from the immediate supervisor to the staff regarding performance, and consequences based on the evaluation (Burgio, 1994).

In the home setting, the caregiver should use a voiding record to document the toileting events and note whether the person was incontinent at the time of toileting. If incontinence worsens or does not improve, the individual should be checked for changes in medical and functional conditions and for other causes of transient incontinence.

Electrical Stimulation

Electrical stimulation has been used in physical therapy for many years. Electrical stimulation for pelvic floor weakness is defined as "the application of electrical current to stimulate the pelvic viscera or their nerve supply" (ICS Committee, 1992, p. 102). The exact mechanism of electrical stimulation is not completely understood. Its purpose is to invoke a therapeutic response from the reflex arc in the sacral area of the spinal cord via surface or percutaneous electrodes or implants. The mode of stimulation can be one time only, continuous, phasic, or intermittent. Electrical stimulation is not appropriate for an individual with incontinence due to a complete lower motor neuron lesion, because the required intact reflex arc is absent (ICS Committee, 1992). Electrical stimulation has been used with stress incontinence secondary to weak pelvic muscles and with postprostatectomy incontinence and urge incontinence (Fall & Lindstrom, 1991;

Laycock, 1994). If there is no reduction in symptoms in four or five sessions the treatment should be discontinued (Davis, 1995).

SURGICAL INTERVENTIONS

The AHCPR Clinical Practice Guideline Update Panel for Urinary Incontinence in Adults recommends surgical intervention only after a concise and detailed evaluation of the incontinence is performed (Fantl et al., 1996). The evaluation will include a correlation of the anatomical and physiological findings with the surgical plan, weighing of the risks and benefits of the surgical procedure, and an estimation of the effects of the surgery on the individual's quality of life.

Men with Overflow and Stress Incontinence

One of the most common urological causes of urinary incontinence in older men is prostatic hyperplasia. To relieve the obstruction at the bladder outlet caused by the enlarged prostate gland, one of several procedures may be performed.

Balloon dilation of the urethra is used to expand the urethra at the point of constriction. A catheter with an uninflated balloon at its end is passed through to the prostatic urethra to the area narrowed by the prostate; the balloon is then inflated to stretch open the urethra. The most common surgical procedure to relieve symptoms due to prostatic hyperplasia is the transurethral resection (TURP). The inner portion of the prostate is removed through an endoscopic instrument passed through the urethra. There is no abdominal scarring with this procedure. Another procedure is the transurethral incision of the prostate (TUIP), whereby the obstruction of the urethra by the prostate is relieved when an endoscopic instrument is passed through the urethra and the physician makes small incisions in the prostate and prostate capsule. An open prostatectomy is another surgical procedure that removes the inner portion of the prostate through a suprapubic or retropubic incision. As discussed in Chapter 3, if the nerves that supply the bladder are disrupted and/or the urethral sphincter is damaged during surgery, or if lesions are present in the spinal cord and/or cerebral cortex from other concomitant conditions, incontinence may persist after surgery. Treatment for postsurgical urinary incontinence, which may be transient or permanent, is dependent on cause.

Periurethral bulking injections have been used to treat men with intrinsic sphincter incompetence. Collagen or a substance known as polytetrafluoroethylene (PTFE) can be injected into the periurethral area to increase urethral compression.

An artificial sphincter to relieve sphincter incompetence after surgical intervention for prostatic hyperplasia can be implanted. Nonsurgical interventions for obstruction due to prostate hyperplasia include avoidance of anticholinergic medications, administration of alpha-adrenergic receptor blockers, suprapubic catheterization, and intermittent catheterization.

Women with Stress Incontinence

For women with stress incontinence secondary to anatomical defects that cause hypermobility of the urethra (such as pelvic floor relaxation or intrinsic sphincter deficiency caused by previous surgery or neurogenic or non-neurogenic factors), there are several surgical interventions that restore the urethral position or increase urethral resistance. Surgical procedures used to reposition the urethra include anterior vaginal repair, retropubic suspension, and needle suspension (Fantl et al., 1996). Surgical procedures to compress the urethra and increase resistance include sling procedures, placement of an artificial sphincter, and periurethral bulking agents. Complications and success rates for each procedure must be discussed with the patient prior to surgery.

PHARMACOLOGICAL INTERVENTIONS

There are several groups of medications used in the treatment of incontinence (see Table 5–2). Prior to the prescription and administration of a medication, the pathophysiology of the incontinence, the mode of action, therapeutic effects, and side effects should be understood. The major sites of medication action are the bladder, trigone and bladder neck, urethra, and prostate (Sourander, 1990) (see Figure 5–1). Although calcium channel blockers are indicated in Figure 5–1, they currently are not recommended in the treatment of detrusor instability (Fantl et al., 1996). Because there can be serious side effects, medications should be used cautiously. Medications should be used in conjunction with a voiding schedule or a behavioral intervention (Fantl et al., 1996).

Alpha-adrenergic receptors are located mainly at the bladder outlet and along the urethra. Alpha-adrenergic receptors when stimulated increase urethral resistance. Beta-adrenergic receptors are located throughout the body of the bladder and when stimulated cause relaxation. Cholinergic receptors are located throughout the bladder and urethra and when stimulated mediate contractions of the bladder. During the storage phase of micturition, the bladder is relaxed and the high urethral resistance keeps the urethra closed, preventing urine from leaking from the bladder into the urethra. Therefore, storage is primarily a sympathetic activity. During emptying of the bladder, however, there is sympathetic inhibition and increased parasympathetic activity, leading to lower urethral resistance and bladder contractions (Yochum, Boyer, & Katz, 1993).

Table 5-2 Medications Used To Treat Urinary Incontinence

Type of Medication	Action	Site of Action	Type of UI	Side Effects
Anticholinergics	Facilitate storage	Bladder wall	Urge	Confusion, Dizziness, Constipation, Blurred vision, Tachycardia, Dry mouth
Bladder relaxants	Facilitate storage	Bladder wall	Urge	Dry mouth, Constipation, Dry skin
Alpha-adrenergic agonists	Facilitate storage	Bladder wall and urethra	Stress	Blood pressure elevation, Insomnia, Anxiety, Tremor, headache, palpitations, cardiac arrhythmias
Tricyclic antidepressants	Facilitate storage	Bladder muscle	Urge	Orthostatic hypotension, Fatigue, Dizziness, Blurred vision, Dry mouth
Estrogens	Facilitate storage	Urethra	Stress	Bleeding, Breast tenderness, Thromboembolism, Neoplasm in estrogen-responsive organs

Anticholinergic Medications

Anticholinergic medications, which decrease bladder contractions and increase bladder capacity, are used to facilitate bladder storage. Therefore, anticholinergics are used in cases of detrusor overactivity that leads to urge incontinence. One of the anticholinergic medications commonly used in the treatment of incontinence

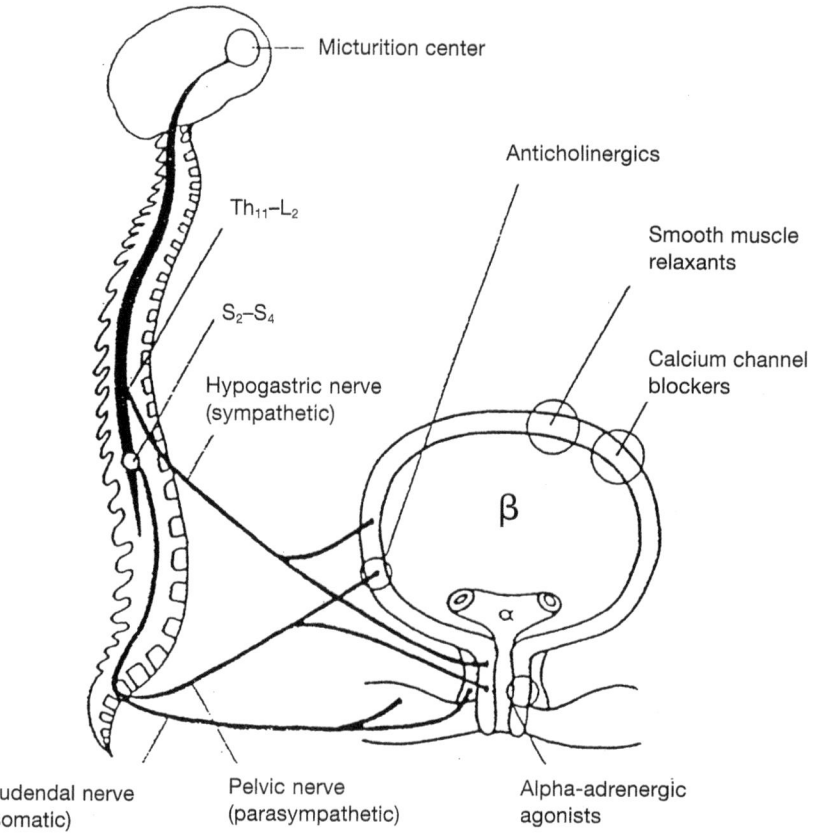

Figure 5–1 Drug Action Sites. *Source:* Reprinted from Sourander, L., Treatment of Urinary Incontinence: The Place of Drugs, *Gerontology*, Vol. 36, Suppl. 2, p. 20, with permission of S Karger AG, © 1990.

---

is propantheline bromide. Some side effects include urinary retention, blurring of the vision, dry mouth, nausea, vomiting, tachycardia, constipation, drowsiness, and confusion. These side effects may be poorly tolerated by older adults. All anticholinergic medications are contraindicated in individuals with narrow-angle glaucoma. Caution must be used in the treatment of detrusor hyperactivity with impaired contractility (DHIC). The administration of anticholinergic medications and/or muscle relaxants could lead to urinary retention.

Smooth Muscle Relaxants

Smooth muscle relaxants with a direct effect on the detrusor are used to facilitate bladder storage and are used to treat urge incontinence. Some medications have anticholinergic and muscle relaxant effects. These include oxybutynin chloride and dicyclomine hydrochloride. Some side effects include dry mouth, dry skin, blurred vision, nausea, and constipation (Fantl et al., 1996).

Tricyclic Antidepressants

Tricyclic antidepressants have several pharmacological mechanisms, including anticholinergic activity and alpha-adrenergic agonist activity. Therefore, they facilitate bladder storage. Imipramine hydrochloride and doxepin hydrochloride have been used in treating noctural incontinence (Fantl et al., 1996). Some side effects include dry mouth, dizziness, and fatigue. Orthostatic hypotension is another reported side effect (Yochum et al., 1993) that could lead to potentially serious consequences such as injurious falls. Tricyclic antidepressants are effective in alleviating depression, which in turn can help the older adult regain continence.

Alpha-Adrenergic Agonists

Alpha-adrenergic receptors are located near the urethral outlet and when stimulated increase urethral resistance. Therefore, medications with an alpha-adrenergic effect facilitate bladder storage for individuals with stress incontinence. Ephedrine, phenylpropanolamine, and pseudoephedrine have been used to treat stress incontinence. Some side effects that may exclude older adults from taking these medications include elevated blood pressure, anxiety, tremor, insomnia, palpitations, headache, and cardiac arrhythmias.

Estrogens

Estrogen receptors are located in the female urethra and trigone. With the fall of circulating estrogens associated with menopause, urogenital atrophy occurs that may sometimes lead to urinary symptoms such as dysuria, noctural incontinence, and frequency (Cardozo, 1990). Oral and topical estrogen therapies have been used to treat stress and urge incontinence in women. It has been postulated that the administration of estrogen may lead to an increased alpha-adrenergic response of the urethra (Fantl et al., 1996). Sometimes estrogens and alpha-adrenergic agonists are used together in postmenopausal women with intrinsic sphincter deficiency. The increase in alpha-adrenergic receptors due to the estrogen therapy and the medication stimulation of the alpha-adrenergic receptors may be more effective than a single medication regimen. Some of the contraindications for estrogen therapy in postmenopausal women include active liver disease, chronic impaired liver function, recent vascular thrombosis, breast cancer, endometrial carcinoma, and unexplained vaginal bleeding (Marshburn & Carr, 1994). Women should be carefully screened for medical conditions that would prohibit estrogen therapy.

VOIDING MANEUVERS

When behavioral, surgical, and pharmacological interventions are not appropriate to facilitate bladder emptying, voiding maneuvers can be used. The International Continence Society Committee on Standardisation of Terminology (1992) states that the aim of voiding maneuvers is to "achieve complete bladder emptying at low intravesical pressure" (p. 104). These techniques can be noninvasive (Credé and Valsalva maneuvers, anal dilatation, suprapubic tapping) or invasive (intermittent, suprapubic, or indwelling catheterization).

Noninvasive voiding techniques can be combined with behavioral interventions such as teaching the individual to void at specific times (scheduled toileting) and voiding while sitting upright and leaning slightly forward. The Credé and Valsalva maneuvers increase abdominal forces on the bladder. The Credé maneuver involves applying gentle pressure with the hand to the lower abdomen above the symphis pubis while voiding. The Valsalva maneuver involves bearing down gently while positioned to void. Anal dilatation, using a gloved and lubricated finger or small probe, is used with individuals who have an intact sacral reflex arc and those who have suprasacral lesions.

Intermittent catheterization (IC), in and out catheterization, is performed approximately every 3 to 6 hours. Intermittent catheterization (IC) is an appropriate long-term therapy for individuals with chronic urinary retention (Fantl et al., 1996). There may be lower incidence of symptomatic bacteriuria with IC than there is with indwelling catheters (Fantl et al., 1996). Intermittent catheterization also provides the individual freedom from having the constant reminder of the disruption that accompanies the ever-present drainage bag used with indwelling catheterization. Many individuals, including older adults, can be taught how to self-catheterize. Candidates for this treatment must be cognitively intact and unencumbered by major physical disabilities that would prevent insertion of the catheter.

Suprapubic catheterization involves a surgical incision in the abdomen to pass a catheter into the bladder. It may be used as a short- or long-term therapy of urinary drainage, but it is contraindicated in people with chronic detrusor instability or intrinsic sphincter deficiency (Fantl et al., 1996). Suprapubic catheterization is preferable over indwelling catheterization for long-term bladder drainage in order to avoid urethral complications associated with long-term usage of an urethral catheter. However, caregivers must be educated regarding proper management strategies.

Indwelling catheters should be used only when there are no other options for alternative therapy. The complications of long-term catheterization are well known: symptomatic bacteriuria, obstruction, stone formation, and renal involvement (Warren, 1995). Catheterization is further discussed in Chapter 8.

TREATMENT OF FUNCTIONAL INCONTINENCE

Impaired mobility, because it limits access to toilet facilities, has been implicated as a cause of functional incontinence (Jirovec & Wells, 1990). Limited mobility secondary to arthritis is a common condition in older adults. Stiff and painful joints discourage an individual from exercising or increasing his or her tolerance for exercise. Therefore, limited mobility can cause incontinence simply because the toilet remains inaccessible. Besides treating the underlying cause of the limited mobility, the treatment regimen for urinary incontinence includes providing accessible and spacious toilet facilities, making available and helping the older adult to utilize appropriate devices to enhance mobility (e.g., walkers, canes, and properly fitting shoes), and planning activities in close proximity of a bathroom.

Attractive, loose, easy-to-remove clothing can help to overcome limited manual dexterity. The use of Velcro fasteners, snaps instead of buttons, wrap skirts, extra fullness in dresses, and Velcro trouser openings can facilitate rapid removal to prevent soiling from incontinence.

To enhance functioning in activities of daily living, sensory deficits should be corrected. Older adults who are unable to see or hear accurately receive impaired messages from others and the environment. This can cause misinterpretation and incorrect or inappropriate responses by the older adult. Correction of the deficits includes not only wearing eyeglasses and hearing aids but also proper lighting (lighting from several sources rather than one bright source and low glare), easy-to-read signs (large, bold print), and decreased ambient noises (turning down blaring radios and televisions, and reducing the level of conversations among staff members).

Adequate toilet facilities must exist for the older adult. Nonglare lighting; nonskid flooring; provisions for privacy; space to turn around while maneuvering canes and walkers; and a place to rest a cane, pocketbook, or purse are necessary factors in securing appropriate arrangements for older adults. Besides good lighting and privacy, the toilet area should be warm and well ventilated. A call system to obtain assistance from the staff should be readily accessible.

Toilet seats should be raised to prevent excessive flexion of the hips and to facilitate rising from the toilet. Armrests and security rails should be firmly attached and in easy reach of the older adult. Again, loose-fitting and easy-to-remove clothing helps to facilitate continence.

Urinary incontinence can occur when physical restraints are used. The use of physical restraints should be eliminated unless a medical condition necessitates their use, and they must be used only under a physician's order. The older adult should be under constant surveillance while the restraints are in place. Explanations must be given for why restraints are being used, whether or not the caregiver thinks that the older adult is capable of understanding the explanation. Toilet facilities should be offered at least every 2 hours. Privacy should be provided while the individual is using the toilet or toilet substitute. Before restraints are implemented, the benefits of their use must be carefully weighed against the hazards. As soon as the individual's medical condition permits, physical restraint should be discontinued.

TREATMENT OF TRANSIENT INCONTINENCE

The choice of treatment depends on the causative factor. The caregiver may use DIAPPERS, DRIP (see Chapter 3), and the RAP component of the Minimum Data Set (described in Chapter 4) to assess the causes of transient incontinence and to initiate appropriate treatment. Some of the most common treatments of transient incontinence follow.

Urinary Tract Infections

If a urinary tract infection is discovered during assessment, appropriate antibiotics are prescribed as indicated by the sensitivity report accompanying the urine culture results. Antiseptic medications, such as pyridium, may be prescribed as well. Cranberry juice has been proven effective in treating urinary tract infections caused by some strains of *Escherichia coli* (Avorn et al., 1994). Adequate oral hydration (30 ml/kg of body weight daily) (Lipschitz, 1992), regular toileting to prevent stasis of urine, and good hygiene habits are fundamental parts of the treatment of incontinence caused by urinary tract infection (UTI).

Patient education is an integral element in treatment. Sexually active women with a history of urge incontinence from urinary tract infections should be counseled to void immediately after intercourse, wash hands before touching genitalia, and increase oral fluid intake.

Incontinence caused by bladder stones or bladder tumors may require surgical intervention.

Fecal Impaction

The best treatment of fecal impaction is prevention. In the institutional setting, keeping and evaluating a daily record of bowel movements is one way to prevent constipation and impaction. A person who gives a history of persistent use of laxatives, limited mobility, diabetes mellitus, low-fiber diet, poor fluid intake, and medications with constipating side effects is at risk for being constipated, and if left untreated, impacted. Symptomatic constipation is defined as "two or fewer bowel movements a week, of which 25% involve straining" (Minaker & Harari, 1995).

Bowel management protocols involve setting the same time every day for evacuation, drinking fluids with most of them ingested prior to 6 p.m. to avoid nocturia, physical activity, and a high-fiber diet (Smith, Newman, & Blackwood, 1992). Fiber should be added to the diet gradually to avoid cramping and excess flatulence. Bulk laxatives, such as psyllium, are recommended for constipation in the elderly (Minaker & Harari, 1995).

Delirium

Delirium, an acute confusional state, must be very carefully assessed for its causes. Signs of delirium include disorientation, delusions, illusions, vivid hallucinations, and disturbances in the sleep-wake cycle (Jarvik, Lavretsky, & Neshkes, 1992). Many times, delirium may be a sign of infection in an older person (Breitenbucher, 1990). Some kind of change is the cause of the acute confusional state. By proceeding through a systematic assessment of physiological, psychosocial, and environmental factors, including new medications, the alteration causing the delirium can usually be discovered. While the confusional state persists, scheduled toileting and use of toilet substitutes should be employed. The caregiver should never assume or let the older adult and family assume that incontinence is a permanent condition.

Medications

Certain medications can contribute significantly to the development of urinary incontinence. In order to eliminate this cause of incontinence, caregivers must be knowledgeable about the actions and side effects of drugs prescribed for older adults. Fast-acting diuretics such as furosemide can cause incontinence due to the rapid filling of the bladder and the increased need to void. Administering the drug early in the day when the older adult is active, physically and mentally, can decrease episodes of incontinence during sleep or when physically distant from toilet facilities. By being knowledgeable about a medication's onset of action and its duration, the nurse can alert the staff to offer accessible toilet facilities to the individual throughout the day.

Decreasing the use of hypnotics to promote sleep can help to decrease nocturnal incontinence. Warm baths, back rubs, warm milk, and following a consistent nighttime ritual are effective means of relaxing the individual and facilitating sleep. Nighttime can be a lonely and stressful time for older adults. Being a caring listener, assuaging unwarranted fears through reassurance, and being physically present can help the individual fall asleep without the aid of a drug.

Older adults taking certain medications for treatment of hypertension are at risk for urinary retention, which can contribute to incontinence. To avoid complications, a record of fluids ingested and urinary output helps to alert the staff to fluid imbalance. The older adult should be encouraged to assume the natural positions for voiding (standing and sitting), and to express urine manually using the Credé maneuver to facilitate bladder emptying. Patient teaching about any treatment is important to the success of the program but, as with any drug therapy, the individual should be alerted to side and untoward effects of all medications (including over-the-counter medications) and be encouraged to report any unusual symptoms to the nurse or physician.

TREATMENT SETTINGS

Long-Term Care Setting

Incontinence is a significant problem in the long-term care setting. As discussed in Chapter 3, approximately 50% of long-term care residents are incontinent. After assessing incontinence using the Minimum Data Set and Resident Assessment Profile, treatment options should be considered. There are several common elements to all the treatments used in long-term care. These include communication between the older adult and caregiver, hydration, prevention of skin breakdown, control of odor, and habit formation (Fowler, Ouslander, & Papen, 1990).

Daily fluid intake, through ingested fluids, in food, and from water produced by metabolism is approximately 2,100 to 2,800 ml (Williams, 1989). The daily water requirement is 30 ml/kg of body weight (Lipschitz, 1992). Because thirst sensation may be decreased in older adults, fluids should be offered throughout the day, especially with adults who cannot independently feed themselves. Skin care is critical to all older adults. Aging skin is less vascular and thinner than young skin and may be vulnerable to breakdown, especially in skin over bony prominences exposed to unrelieved pressure (Clinical Practice Guideline Panel, 1992). Perineal care with a terry washcloth and soap can cause dry, irritated skin (Jeter, 1992). Special washes that cleanse and protect from drying of the skin are preferable to soap. Moisturizers and barriers that repel urine and stool can also protect the skin. Skin care, as all care, should be individualized. Selection of skin care products should be based on a careful assessment of the person's overall condition and the condition of the skin. A broad spectrum antifungal cream should be used for yeast infections (Fowler et al., 1990).

The best prevention of odor is prevention of an incontinent episode. However, if an incontinent episode should occur, the person, soiled clothing, and furniture should be cleaned immediately. Commercial preparations are available to help control odor.

All behavioral therapies used in long-term care facilities involve changing behaviors and forming new habits. Once the new behavior is selected, e.g., continence during the day, antecedents that will evoke that behavior (verbal prompts to use the toilet, assistance to the bathroom) and consequences (increased participation in social activities, attractive undergarments and clothing, decreased use of absorbent products) must be determined prior to the implementation of new programs that involve feedback, reinforcement, and consistent implementation.

The outcome of the intervention also must be considered prior to implementation. Exhibit 5–2 displays four possible outcomes. Independent continence, dependent continence, and social continence were first described by Fonda (1990). Partial continence was developed to describe the outcomes of improved continence without achieving total continence after a behavioral therapy was started (Palmer, 1995).

Independent continence refers to the individual who is able to maintain continence without assistance. Interventions that may support an independently continent individual include environmental modifications to keep access to the toilet optimal, exercise programs that promote fitness and mobility, the use of a limited course of topical estrogen cream to treat atrophic vaginitis, and pelvic muscle exercise to maintain pelvic floor tone.

Dependent continence refers to individuals who are kept continent solely through the efforts of the nursing staff. These individuals are usually cognitively or functionally impaired and require assistance to use the toilet in a timely manner.

Exhibit 5–2 Continence Outcomes

		Urinary Continence	Urinary Incontinence
Need for physical help for timely access to toilet	No	Independent continence	Chronic management to attain social continence
	Yes	Dependent continence	Behavior and combination of interventions to achieve partial incontinence

During assessment, these individuals have the ability to delay voiding and usually have a high rate of dryness prior to implementation of a program of regular toileting.

Environmental modifications and use of toilet substitutes to increase access to the toilet facilities are important to maintaining continence. Several behavioral therapies previously described are appropriate as well, and should be selected based on the assessment of the individual and desired outcomes. These therapies include bladder training, scheduled toileting, and prompted voiding.

As mentioned earlier, because of the importance of providing the behavioral therapy in a consistent manner, staff training and management systems are suggested (Burgio & Burgio, 1990). Staff training should consist of a review of the anatomy of the urinary tract, the causes of transient and established incontinence, the outcomes and objectives of the treatment, and the performance expectations of the staff. One method of providing staff feedback about the effectiveness of the prompted voiding is a quality control method developed by Schnelle (1991). Using this method, a bladder record is kept for 3 days and the number of continent and incontinent events are recorded. The average and standard deviation of incontinent events are calculated, and this information is used as a quality indicator. Another method of providing staff feedback about the effectiveness of the therapy, prompted voiding, the Behavioral Supervision Model, is employed (Burgio, 1994). This consists of defining the responsibilities of the staff for the prompted voiding intervention, staff feedback regarding performance in carrying out the intervention, and consequences based on job performance (Burgio, 1994).

Partial continence refers to the individual continence pattern in which there is improved dryness. The individual is dry part of the time due to the effects of the nursing staff to help the individual to retain urine in the bladder until toilet facilities are reached. The individual has mostly continent voids, but has, even with behavioral interventions, wet episodes. These individuals on assessment exhibit the potential for improving or maintaining dryness but cannot attain total continence. There will be a different level of dryness for each individual. The success of the intervention is based on the difference between the individual's level of dryness prior to the intervention and the level of dryness after the intervention was started. Environmental modifications and use of toilet substitutes are important components of interventions for partially continent residents. Behavioral therapies include prompted voiding, habit training, and scheduled toileting.

Social continence is achieved only through the use of containment measures, such as absorbent products. The goal is to keep the individual dry, odor free, and socially acceptable. Since the individual is not capable of retaining urine within the body until it is time to empty the bladder, urine is retained on the body via external devices (condom catheters) or by using absorbent products. Chapter 8 discusses these interventions in detail.

Home Care Setting

Many of the treatments in the long-term care setting are appropriate for the home care setting. A family caregiver may be the individual responsible for carrying out the interventions; therefore, the relationship between the caregiver and patient, the caregiver's ability and desire to implement treatment, and the caregiver's understanding of the outcomes and objectives of the selected treatment must be assessed (Appleby, 1995). The environment should be modified, if possible, to provide easy access to the bathroom. The voiding record is a helpful measure of the effectiveness of the interventions in improving continence.

Care of the indwelling catheter in the home consists of education of the caregiver. Topics for education include anatomy and physiology of the urinary tract, information about the size and type of the catheter, care of the catheter, and possible complications (Fiers, 1995). See Chapter 8 for more discussion of indwelling catheter care.

Acute Care Setting

Incontinence in the acute care setting may be established or transient. Caregivers should attempt to prevent deterioration of continence status during the hospital stay. Using scheduled toileting, providing toilet substitutes, assessing for and eliminating the causes of transient incontinence, and providing public education about incontinence and community referrals for continence services are some treatment options available to the acute care caregiver. Indwelling catheters should be avoided if possible.

CONCLUSION

The treatment of incontinence is complex. It is based on the findings collected during assessment, along with the needs and concerns of the older adult. Selection of the appropriate treatment should include mutual goal setting with the older adult. Education regarding the advantages, disadvantages, and outcome should be provided to the older adult with any treatment modality. Treatments range from sophisticated surgical procedures to everyday common sense. The cornerstone of the approach to treatment is the realistic optimism of the health care team and the committed determination to alleviate the physical and emotional distress of urinary incontinence.

REFERENCES

Appleby, S. (1995). A home health perspective on the management of urinary incontinence. *Journal of Wound, Ostomy, and Continence Nursing, 22*, 145–152.

Avorn, J., Monane, M., Gurwitz, J., Glynn, R., Choodnovskly, I., & Lipsitz, L. (1994). Reduction of bacteriuria and pyuria after ingestion of cranberry juice. *Journal of the American Medical Association, 271*, 751–754.

Breitenbucher, R. (1990). UTI: Managing the most common nursing home infection. *Geriatrics, 45*, 68–75.

Burgio, L. (1994). Improving caregiver compliance with behavioral interventions. Paper presented at the meeting of UCLA/JHA Anna & Harry Borun Center for Gerontological Research, Atlanta, GA.

Burgio, L., & Burgio, K. (1990). Institutional staff training and management: A review of the literature and a model for geriatric, long-term care facilities. *International Journal of Aging and Human Development, 30*, 287–302.

Burgio, K., & Engel, B. (1990). Biofeedback-assisted behavioral training for elderly men and women. *Journal of the American Geriatrics Society, 38*, 338–340.

Burgio, K., Ives, D., Locher, J., Arena, V., & Kuller, L. (1994). Treatment seeking for urinary incontinence in older adults. *Journal of the American Geriatrics Society, 42*, 208–212.

Cardozo, L. (1990). Role of estrogens in the treatment of female urinary incontinence. *Journal of the American Geriatrics Society, 38*, 326–328.

Clinical Practice Guideline Panel. (1992). *Clinical practice guideline: Pressure ulcers in adults: Prediction and prevention* (AHCPR Pub. No. 92-0047). Rockville, MD: Agency for Health Care Policy and Research, Public Health Service, U.S. Department of Health and Human Services.

Colling, J., Ouslander, J., Hadley, B., Eisch, J., & Campbell, E. (1992). The effects of patterned urge-response toileting (PURT) on urinary incontinence among nursing home residents. *Journal of the American Geriatrics Society, 40*, 135–141.

Coxe, J. (1994). Assessment for biofeedback and behavioral therapy for urinary incontinence. *Urologic Nursing, 14*(3), 82–84.

Davis, V. (1995). Electrical stimulation: Does nursing have a role in the treatment of adult urinary incontinence? *Urologic Nursing, 15*(20), 56–60.

Fall, M., & Lindstrom, S. (1991). Electrical stimulation: A physiological approach to the treatment of urinary incontinence. *Urologic Clinics of North America, 18*, 393–407.

Fantl, A., Wyman, J., McClish, D., Harkins, S., Elswick, R., Taylor, J., & Hadley, E. (1991). Efficacy of bladder training in older women with urinary incontinence. *Journal of the American Medical Association, 265*, 609–613.

Fantl, J.A., Newman, D.K., & Colling, J. et al. (1996). *Urinary incontinence in adults: Acute and chronic management. Clinical practice guideline no. 2, 1996 update.* (AHCPR Pub. No. 96-0692). Rockville, MD: Agency for Health Care Policy and Research, Public Health Service, U.S. Department of Health and Human Services.

Fiers, S. (1995). Management of the long-term indwelling catheter in the home setting. *Journal of Wound, Ostomy and Continence Nursing, 22*, 140–144.

Flynn, L., Cell, P., & Luisi, E. (1994). Effectiveness of pelvic muscle exercises in reducing urge incontinence among community residing elders. *Journal of Gerontological Nursing, 20*(5), 23–27.

Fonda, D. (1990). Improving management of urinary incontinence in geriatric centres and nursing homes. *Australia Clinical Review, 10*, 66–71.

Fowler, E., Ouslander, J., & Papen, J. (1990). Managing incontinence in the nursing home population. *Journal of Enterostomal Therapy, 17*, 77–86.

Housten, K. (1993). Incontinence and the older woman. *Clinics in Geriatric Medicine, 9*(1), 157–171.

International Continence Society Committee on Standardization of Terminology. (1992). Seventh report on the standardization of terminology of lower urinary tract function: Lower urinary tract rehabilitation techniques. *Scandinavian Journal of Urology and Nephrology, 26*.

Jarvik, L., Lavretsky, E., & Neshkes, R. (1992). Dementia and delirium in old age. In J. Brocklehurst, R. Tollis, and T. Fillit (Eds.), *The textbook of geriatric medicine and gerontology* (4th ed.). New York: Churchill Livingstone.

Jeter, K. (1992, June). The special skin care needs of incontinent patients: An ET clinician's view. *Wound and Skin Care*, 90–97.

Jirovec, M., & Wells, T. (1990). Urinary incontinence in nursing home residents with dementia: The mobility-cognition paradigm. *Applied Nursing Research, 3*, 112–117.

Laycock, J. (1994). Pelvic muscle exercises: Physiotherapy for the pelvic floor. *Urologic Nursing, 14*(3), 136–140.

Lipschitz, D. (1992). Nutrition and ageing. In J. Evans & T.F. Williams (Eds.), *Oxford textbook of geriatric medicine.* New York: Oxford University Press.

Marshburn, P., & Carr, B. (1994). The menopause and hormone replacement therapy. In W. Hazard, E. Bierman, J. Blass, W. Ettinger, & J. Hatter (Eds.), *Principles of geriatric medicine and gerontology* (3rd ed.). New York: McGraw-Hill.

Miller, J., Kapser, C., & Sampselle, C. (1994). Review of muscle physiology with application to pelvic muscle exercise. *Urologic Nursing, 14*(3), 92–97.

Minaker, K., & Harari, D. (1995, May 15). Constipation in the elderly. *Hospital Practice*, 67–76.

Newman, D., & Smith, D. (1992). Pelvic muscle reeducation as a nursing treatment for incontinence. *Urologic Nursing, 12*(1), 9–15.

Palmer, M. (1995). A new framework for urinary continence outcomes in institutionalized older adults. Unpublished manuscript.

Palmer, M. (1990). Incontinence in the elderly. In K. Jeter, N. Faller, & C. Norton (Eds.), *Nursing for continence.* Philadelphia: Saunders.

Palmer, M., Bennett, R., Marks, J., McCormick, K., & Engel, B. (1994). Urinary incontinence: A program that works. *Journal of Long-Term Care Administration, 22*(2), 19–25.

Palmer, M., & McCormick, K. (1991). Alterations in elimination: Urinary incontinence. In E. Baines (Ed.), *Perspectives in gerontological nursing.* Thousand Oaks, CA: Sage.

Sale, P., & Wyman, J. (1994). Achievement of goals associated with bladder training by older incontinent women. *Applied Nursing Research, 7*(2), 93–96.

Schnelle, J. (1991). *Managing urinary continence in the elderly.* New York: Springer.

Smith, D., Newman, D., & Blackwood, N. (1992). Urinary incontinence. The unspoken problem. *Office Nurse, 5*(4), 12–20.

Smith, D., & Newman, D. (1994). Basic elements of biofeedback therapy for pelvic muscle rehabilitation. *Urologic Nursing, 14*(3), 130–135.

Sourander, L. (1990). Treatment of urinary incontinence: The place of drugs. *Gerontology, 36*(Suppl.), 19–26.

Tries, J. (1990). Kegel exercises enhanced by biofeedback. *Journal of Enterostomal Therapy, 17*(2), 67–76.

Warren, J. (1995). Guidelines for protecting the patient undergoing long-term urinary catheterization. *Nursing Home Medicine, 3*(5), 95–100.

Wells, T. (1990). Pelvic (floor) muscle exercises. *Journal of the American Geriatrics Society, 38*, 333–337.

Williams, S. (1989). *Nutrition and diet therapy* (6th ed.). St. Louis: Mosby.

Yochum, K., Boyer, J., & Katz, M. (1993). Pharmacologic therapy of incontinence. In R. Bressler & M. Katz (Eds.), *Geriatric pharmacology.* New York: McGraw-Hill.

CHAPTER

6

Psychological Impact

OVERVIEW

The storage and voluntary emptying of urine is a physiological process influenced by social norms. When these norms are violated, there are social and psychological consequences. An important reason to understand these influences is that people's responses, including those of health care providers, to incontinence are rooted in societal expectations, norms, and values. These responses can result in behaviors such as not seeking treatment to providing only palliative rather than rehabilitative treatment.

It has been reported repeatedly in the literature that normal aging does not cause urinary incontinence. Still there is a continuing cultural myth that old age is a time of decline and incompetence, and that incontinence is only one of many signs of this deterioration.

The medical model of a single causative agent and curative approach to disease is an insufficient model for assessing and treating the condition of urinary incontinence (Palmer, 1994). Incontinence is not a disease but a condition, with multiple etiologies; associated factors; and physical, psychological, and social consequences. Therefore, consideration of the psychological aspects of incontinence is necessary when continence promotion strategies are being planned.

The psychological aspects of urinary incontinence for affected older adults, families, and the nursing staff are discussed. This chapter also presents a brief discussion of the historical development of the social norms and influences surrounding sanitation, personal hygiene, and urinary elimination.

HISTORICAL PERSPECTIVE

The current society demand for high levels of personal cleanliness and sanitation is a relatively recent phenomenon. Bathing one's body received scant attention in the world that followed the demise of the pagan Roman Empire. In Europe during the Middle Ages, bathing was viewed as a sinful worldly indulgence. Disposal or removal of excreta from the home or village was an issue of low priority. In fact, the garderobes, or toilets, in the Tower of London were built into the walls with direct openings to the outside. As a result, human wastes drained down the outside walls (Kilroy, 1984). Rivers and streams were used as sewers, and slop buckets were emptied out windows into the streets to the peril of passersby (Figure 6–1). No connection between the spread of disease and sanitation was made until the 19th century.

As the evidence mounted that disease could be prevented through sanitation, the proponents of public health laws were often subjected to scorn and ridicule by those who believed that the spread of disease was God's law. Whereas in many ancient civilizations there were prescribed religious rituals for cleansing the body, washing hands, and removal of excreta (Reynolds, 1974), late 19th century United States and European legislative efforts to enforce proper disposal of excreta and to protect drinking water were considered interfering with God's work. Despite this resistance, the responsibility for sanitation became the responsibility of governments and secular agencies.

However, with the rise of secular sanitation, those who became scorned and ridiculed were not the clean, but rather the uncleaned. Being malodorous or incontinent has become a strong social stigma. A stigmatized person is considered different and less desirable than others (Goffman, 1963). Many people can recall from early school days a child with body odor being mercilessly taunted by classmates and peers. Children who wet their beds are often wrongly subjected to feelings of shame and disgust by parents and siblings, even in well-meaning attempts to stop the behavior.

Voluntary control over one's bowels and bladder is one signal of passage into the society of the adult world. The converse, loss of urinary control, especially in older adults, can mean removal from society and banishment to the world of shameful feelings, rubber sheets, and diapers. Mitteness (1990) noted that incontinence can serve as a signal of the inevitable decline into incompetence that is expected in old age by many cultures. This myth, that incontinence is an expected part of aging, leads to a sense of futility of treatment and the lack of reporting incontinence by older adults to health care providers and, at times, to a failure by health care providers to respond with treatment for the incontinence.

Although voluntary control over one's urinary function is considered a social necessity, it can often be a difficult goal to obtain. Bathrooms in public places are often located in the farthest part of a building, down flights of stairs, or at the end of a long corridor with cryptic pictures (e.g., of hens/roosters; bucks/does) posted

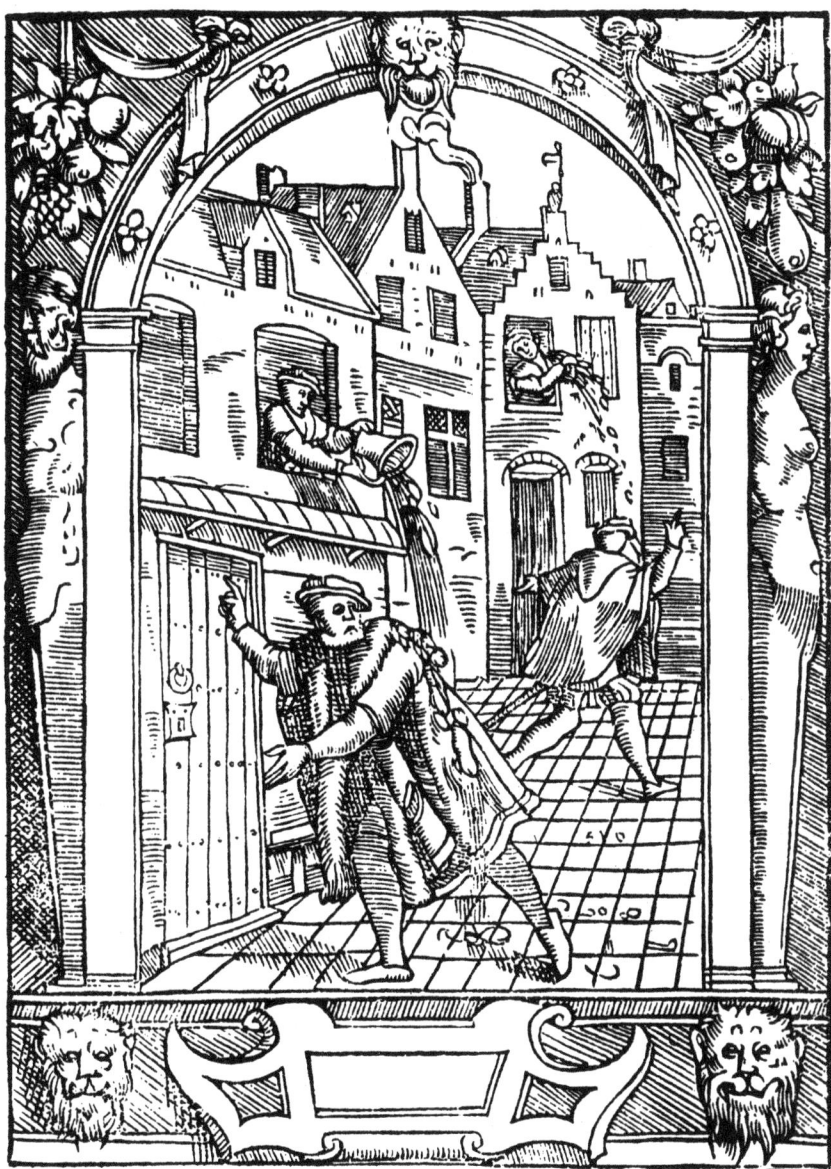

Figure 6–1 A Medieval Street Scene. Courtesy of The Fotomas Index, J.R. Freeman & Co. (Photographers) Ltd., London.

on the doors to denote gender. All too often few commodes are located in women's public restrooms, creating long lines and long waits for access. Public toilet facilities, if allowed to fall into disrepair and states of uncleanliness, are repellent even to those in desperate need of access.

A rather inflexible protocol for public continence exists. One must have not only the desire to void but the ability to locate a bathroom, translate euphemisms on the doors, wait for an available toilet, have the manual dexterity to open and lock doors, undress, change positions, reposition clothes, and wash hands—often having to carry out these activities in places lacking in privacy, space, and cleanliness.

In this context, it is surprising that few services have existed previously to deal effectively with urinary incontinence. Societal priorities must undergo a change so that provisions for continence are considered important and facilitated within society. These values could be operationalized as laundry services for community-dwelling incontinent older adults, fashionable yet easy-to-remove clothing, and architectural designs for the members of society who are not continent and want to remain part of the community. But these services will evolve only through public demand.

PSYCHOLOGICAL IMPACT ON THE OLDER ADULT

To affected older adults, urinary incontinence often represents a loss of control over an especially private bodily function. Older adults have reported feelings of being betrayed by their bodies, and their anger is directed inward (Mitteness, 1987a). As with any loss, expressions of grief, mourning, and depression may be common, especially in people whose incontinence is relatively new. Mitteness (1987a) found that people with long-standing incontinence develop a stoic, matter-of-fact approach to incontinence management, but still suffer acute embarrassment when an incontinent episode occurs.

When the nature of the incontinence is unpredictable, a heightened sense of loss of control may result (Wyman, Harkins, Choi, Taylor, & Fantl, 1987). Rather than risking embarrassment of an "accident," an older adult may decline offers to go out, and stop asking people to visit, consequently losing vital intellectual stimulation and social supports. The lack of a confidant, a serious and frequent problem for the older adult who outlives friends, spouse, and family members, often forces the incontinent older adult to harbor the secret of urinary incontinence alone. The additional stress caused by these bottled-up feelings compounds and heightens the feelings of shame and alienation from society. Mitteness (1992) reported that older adults have little understanding of how their bodies function and do not know whether or not changes are normal. Women, in particular, may be reluctant to discuss incontinence with others, because of a lifelong barrage of messages from the authorities and advertisers that the genital area is unclean and that odors and discharge are unacceptable (Andrist & Maillet, 1992). When incontinence and other disorders occur, feelings of shame and self-blame are often encountered. See Exhibit 6–1 for the psychological impact of urinary incontinence on the older adult.

Many older adults, often with great effort and resourcefulness, have independently controlled their urinary incontinence for many years without the aid of outside resources (Jeter & Wagner, 1990). Some community-living women with urinary incontinence are very successful in developing strategies to preserve their self-esteem and maintain a normal lifestyle (see Exhibit 6–2). These women use measures to prevent accidents and avoid detection by others. Incontinence was seen as a social problem that needed management rather than a medical one that could be treated (Dowd, 1991).

Exhibit 6–1 Psychological Impact of Urinary Incontinence

Older Adult	Families	Health Care Providers
Anxiety	Burdensome	Avoidance
Depression	Tiring	Incontinence care seen as time consuming, frustrating, aesthetically displeasing
Helplessness	Difficult	
Sadness	Anger	
Pessimism	Resentment	
Low self-esteem		Less sympathetic and more blaming
Stress		
Insecurity		
Anger		
Feeling undignified		
Ashamed		
Self-blame		
Impatient		
Feeling of being an outcast		
Uncomfortable due to dampness		
Embarrassment		
Socially disruptive		
Loss of control		
Worry		
Social isolation		
Mourning		
Futility		

Exhibit 6–2 Self-Care System To Meet the Self-Care Requisites Related to Urinary Incontinence (UI)

Self-Care Requisites Related to UI	Self-Care System
Prevention of threat to self-esteem	Stage 1: Being in charge a. effective continence care b. being prepared c. planning
Provision of care for products of urinary elimination	Stage 2: Accepting UI a. confidence in care routine b. best it can be c. minimizing
Promotion of normalcy	Stage 3: Normalizing a. routinizing b. desired lifestyle

Source: Reprinted from Dowd, T., Discovering Older Women's Experience of Urinary Incontinence, *Research in Nursing and Health*, Vol. 14, p. 185, with permission of John Wiley & Sons, © 1990.

All too often a hospitalization, an acute illness, or a change in routine can result in having another person detect the incontinence. The fear of discovery is very real. It has been reported that urinary incontinence is one reason for institutionalization of an older adult (Fantl, Newman, & Colling et al., 1996), and many older adults have anecdotal evidence of this fact. Therefore, it is not surprising that an older adult would be reluctant to reveal disruptions in urine control, deny urine leakage, and refuse to discuss treatment modalities with health care providers. The mere thought of sharing this knowledge or having the incontinence exposed may fill an older adult with shame and dread. As mentioned in Chapter 2, one of the dictionary definitions of incontinence connotes immorality and moral looseness. The word itself may be offensive to some, invoking anger, denial, or refusal to discuss the issue at all. It is imperative that health care providers understand the psychological impact of these fears of exposure and vulnerability when urinary incontinence is discovered during history taking or upon physical examination. Often older adults use definitions for incontinence that differ from those of health care providers (Ory, Wyman, & Yu, 1986). Mitteness (1987b) found that older adults living in senior citizen housing did not consider urine loss that did not wet clothing or bed linens as incontinence. Only when the incontinent episode was of sufficient quantity to be detected by others was it considered to be incontinence.

The shame of being incontinent can cause an older adult to retreat further into depths of an existing mental illness or cognitive impairment. By not being "all there," how can one be responsible for wetting oneself? Finally, out of hopelessness an incontinent older adult can assume an attitude of resignation. Especially in an environment where there is little support to maintain independence and where expectations of staff for incontinent behavior exist, a self-fulfilling prophecy occurs and a terrible cycle of shame, incontinence, and reinforced shame is perpetuated. The hopelessness of this scenario can render the older adult emotionally broken and unable to make attempts to regain continence or dignity (Newman, 1962).

The individual with poor lifelong habits regarding personal hygiene may not find incontinent behavior as shameful as would a habitually—even compulsively—clean person (Helps, 1977). For other individuals, proper elimination of waste products may be viewed not so much as a private act but one of personal control and nonconformity to societal demands. Although a rare occurrence, an incontinent act may be performed by these individuals as a way to defy societal values and exhibit control, however inappropriate, over one's life. The psychological effect of this type of behavior is the alienation and distancing of all social supports by willfully deviating from societal norms (Schwartz & Stanton, 1950; Schreter, 1979).

The location of the individual (community versus institution), general health status, functional ability, presence of other illnesses or conditions (including fecal incontinence), length of time incontinent, and severity and frequency of incontinence all may play an important role in the psychological impact of incontinence. For example, Herzog, Fultz, Brock, Brown, and Diokno (1988) found with a large sample of community-dwelling older adults that incontinence was weakly associated with depression, low satisfaction with life, and negative affect. They concluded that these findings may be related to overall poor health status and not solely to the incontinence. Earlier, Simons (1985) found that incontinence did not affect self-concept in a small group of community-dwelling women. Nevertheless, health care providers must use sensitive questions about the impact of incontinence when discussing this condition with older adults.

Standardized questionnaires about the psychological impact of incontinence are available to clinicians and researchers. Norton (1982) described a 17-item, self-administered questionnaire that assessed the effects of incontinence on physical health, mental well-being, and social and personal relations of community-dwelling women. Wyman et al. (1987) adapted this questionnaire in the creation of the Incontinence Impact Questionnaire. It is a 26-item questionnaire, divided into three categories: self-perception, activities of daily living, and social interactions. For institutionalized women, Yu, Kaltreider, Hu, Igou, and Craighead (1989) developed the Incontinence Stress Questionnaire-Patient (ISQ-P), a 36-item, Likert-scale instrument that can be read aloud while the individual holds and reads along on a large-print copy. This scale measures three factors: depressive, aesthetic/somatic, and social. Ouslander and Abelson (1990) reported eight questions asked of outpatients to determine their perceptions of the impact of incontinence on their lives. Burgio, Ives, Locher, Arena, and Kuller (1994) described a 10-point impact scale that asked how incontinence affected feelings and activities.

PSYCHOLOGICAL IMPACT ON THE FAMILIES

Family members have reported that providing continence care is a burdensome task (Flaherty, Miller, & Coe, 1992). Those who provide care to an incontinent older adult at home, especially an older adult incontinent of both urine and stool, describe the tasks as tiring, difficult, and upsetting (Noelker, 1987). Until recently there has been little information available to family members regarding the care of incontinent older adults, limited types of supplies, and little home health care support. The lack of appropriate resources creates a feeling of frustration and a sense of aloneness for an already burdened family member. As energy and health of the family caregiver flags, depressive symptoms can appear (Flaherty et al., 1992). As the condition becomes established and/or worsens, soiled clothing, rugs, and furniture can rapidly turn a household into a living nightmare for both the incontinent older adult and the family.

The experience of seeing a person once able to perform private bodily functions no longer capable of doing so causes great distress and sadness. A process of grieving occurs for the loss of the older adult's independence. Adult children speak with irony and sadness of the role reversal: "Who would have thought at 57 years old I'd have another baby—my mother!" This change in family dynamics can have a profound impact on the relationship between the older adult and the family member. Without adequate social and physical support and confidants, a family member can experience a sense of alienation from the rest of society and express or repress feelings of resentment toward the older adult and toward other family members not directly involved in providing care.

Previous family dynamics and ways of coping must be explored with the family member as health care providers attempt to intervene. Old wounds in the form of unresolved conflicts, both parental and sibling, can present barriers to solving the problems at hand. Family members have many feelings to sort through, including feelings toward the older adult, aging itself, and a conflicting sense of responsibility to both self and others. Urinary incontinence places a significant physical demand on the caregiver. The psychological impact on a family member adds to that burden.

Family members of institutionalized incontinent older adults may feel a need to deny the behavior or to blame the incontinence on the staff. "Mother wasn't like this when she came in here" is not an unusual comment to hear in a long-term care facility. Sometimes, this indictment is deserved by the staff. However, in most instances the family member is not able to accept that a physical disruption within the older adult is responsible for the condition.

Repugnance for the incontinent act may spill over and create repugnance for the incontinent adult. In an attempt to decrease this source of anxiety, the family member may try to create emotional and physical distance.

PSYCHOLOGICAL IMPACT ON THE NURSING STAFF

A paradox exists in Western society; continence and sanitation are highly desirable, but the occupations designed to provide and maintain these conditions are not. Throughout history a stigma has always existed for those who are responsible for removing excreta and maintaining sanitary conditions. The nursing profession is caught in this paradox. Despite nursing's attempt to gain high professional status among other health care workers and the public, the image of the nurse with bedpan in hand persists.

Nurses, as members of society, often reflect societal beliefs and prejudices regarding personal hygiene and incontinence (Wolf, 1986). Besides feeling a personal repugnance toward soiled clothing and body parts, the nursing staff's awareness and internalization of the low opinion held by society of those who work with excreta may foster low self-esteem and morale. In one study, one third of the nurses responding to a survey reported feeling depressed about their work (Yu & Kaltreider, 1987). Nursing staff members as professional caregivers are generally considered to have less emotional involvement with the incontinent patient than do family members. However, nursing staff members sometimes do form strong bonds with their patients and develop low morale and frustration over their incontinent patients.

Withdrawal may be the strategy used by nursing staff in an attempt to deal with the anxiety and frustration that their patients' incontinent behavior creates. Open discussion to facilitate exploration of these feelings is one of the first steps to be taken to define the anxiety. However, when polled about problems on the nursing units or topics for in-service classes, staff members rarely list urinary incontinence (Yu et al., 1991). The hopeless acceptance of incontinence can make it into a nonproblem. Wellings (1988) found that resignation and apathy toward incontinence inevitably turned into demoralization by the staff.

The culture of the nursing home is one that is resistant to change (Wagner & Colling, 1993). Routine rounds can occur to check and change beds without any thought being given to arresting or reversing incontinent behavior. Staff members unwittingly convey the acceptance of incontinence to the incontinent older adult, who in turn perceives the acceptance as positive reinforcement for the incontinent behavior. This is especially true on nursing units where the only staff-patient interactions involve task-oriented activity by the staff. The incontinent older adult correctly perceives that the only way to get attention, albeit cursory physical attention, is through being incontinent.

Staff members who derive a benign sense of satisfaction or a sense of resignation from bathing and applying clean sheets or clothes should examine the source of these feelings. The following three questions should be asked individually or in group discussion:

1. Does my satisfaction or resignation stem from the dependency of the incontinent older adult on the caregiver?
2. Is my satisfaction or resignation derived from observing the incontinent individual's attempt to adapt to the situation with a sense of hopelessness?
3. Am I only making the best of the situation instead of seeking viable alternatives?

Whether the staff member expresses extreme frustration, benign satisfaction, silent resignation, or ambivalence in the care of the incontinent older adult, the feelings must be explored, and basic issues regarding attitudes toward aging, incontinence, personal hygiene, and dependency must be examined and addressed. In-service classes, team conferences, and staff meetings can serve as forums for discussions of these feelings.

When surveyed, nurses believe that continence programs improve patient care (Palmer, 1995). They also report that information is the most important factor in setting up a continence program. Therefore, apparent indifference to incontinence may be a symptom of a lack of information about the normal changes with age, the functioning of the urinary tract, and the pathophysiology of incontinence. Although this education is necessary, research has shown that it is not sufficient to change staff behavior (Campbell, Knight, Benson, & Colling, 1991). It is essential to have an articulate administrative philosophy of continence promotion that translates into meaningful policies for individualized continence care.

CONCLUSION

Besides having a physical impact on older adults, families, and health care providers, urinary incontinence creates a wide gamut of emotional responses. Each individual comes with deeply ingrained social, familial, and personal attitudes. Awareness of the complex nature of the psychological responses and the interdependency of personal response with the more global societal view helps to clarify the needs and expectations of the incontinent older adult, family member, and health care provider. From this understanding comes empathic realistic plans of care and goals of treatment for incontinent older adults.

REFERENCES

Andrist, L., & Maillet, A. (1992). Vulvovaginal conditions: Social, psychological, and sexual considerations. *Nurse Practitioner Forum, 3*, 181–184.

Burgio, K., Ives, D., Locher, J., Arena, V., & Kuller, L. (1994). Treatment seeking for urinary incontinence in older adults. *Journal of the American Geriatrics Society, 42*, 208–212.

Campbell, E., Knight, M., Benson, M., & Colling, J. (1991). Effect of an incontinence training program on nursing home staff's knowledge, attitudes, and behavior. *Gerontologist, 31*, 788–793.

Dowd, T. (1991). Discovering older women's experience of urinary incontinence. *Research in Nursing and Health, 14*, 179–186.

Fantl, J.A., Newman, D.K., & Colling, J. et al. (1996). *Urinary incontinence in adults: Acute and chronic management. Clinical practice guideline no. 2, 1996 update.* (AHCPR Pub. No. 96-0692). Rockville, MD: Agency for Health Care Policy and Research, Public Health Service, U.S. Department of Health and Human Services.

Flaherty, J., Miller, D., & Coe, R. (1992). Impact on caregivers of supporting urinary function in noninstitutionalized, chronically ill seniors. *Gerontologist, 32*, 541–545.

Goffman, E. (1963). *Stigma*. Englewood Cliffs, NJ: Prentice Hall.

Helps, E. (1977). Diseases of the urinary system. *British Medical Journal, 2*, 754–757.

Herzog, A., Fultz, N., Brock, B., Brown, M., & Diokno, A. (1988). Urinary incontinence and psychological distress among older adults. *Psychology and Aging, 3*, 115–121.

Jeter, K., & Wagner, D. (1990). Incontinence in the American home: A survey of 36,500 people. *Journal of the American Geriatrics Society, 38*, 379–383.

Kilroy, R. (1984). *The compleat loo*. London: Victor Gollancz.

Mitteness, L. (1987a). So what do you expect when you're 85? Urinary incontinence in late life. In J. Roth & P. Conrad (Eds.), *Research in the sociology of health care* (Vol. 6, pp. 177–219). Greenwich, CT: JAI Press.

Mitteness, L. (1987b). The management of urinary incontinence by community-living elderly. *Gerontologist, 27*, 185–193.

Mitteness, L. (1990). Knowledge and beliefs about urinary incontinence in adulthood and old age. *Journal of the American Geriatrics Society, 38*, 374–378.

Mitteness, L. (1992). Social aspects of urinary incontinence in the elderly. *AORN Journal, 52*, 731–737.

Newman, J. (1962, June 30). Old folks in wet beds. *British Medical Journal*, 1824–1827.

Noelker, L. (1987). Incontinence in elderly cared for by family. *Gerontologist, 27*, 194–200.

Norton, C. (1982). The effects of urinary incontinence in women. *International Rehabilitation Medicine, 4*, 9–14.

Ory, M., Wyman, J., & Yu, L. (1986). Psychological factors in urinary incontinence. *Clinics in Geriatric Medicine, 2*, 657–671.

Ouslander, J., & Abelson, S. (1990). Perceptions of urinary incontinence among elderly outpatients. *Gerontologist, 30*, 369–372.

Palmer, M. (1994). A health promotion perspective of urinary continence. *Nursing Outlook, 42*(4), 163–169.

Palmer, M. (1995). Nurses' knowledge and beliefs about continence programs in long-term care. *Journal of Advanced Nursing, 21*, 1065–1072.

Reynolds, R. (1974). *Cleanliness & godliness.* New York: Harcourt Brace Jovanovich.

Schreter, C. (1979). Clinical note: Incontinence on the street. *Gerontologist, 19*, 509–511.

Schwartz, M., & Stanton, A. (1950). A social psychological study of incontinence. *Psychiatry, 13*, 399–416.

Simons, J. (1985). Does incontinence affect your client's self-concept? *Journal of Gerontological Nursing, 11*(6), 37–40.

Wagner, A., & Colling, J. (1993). Resistance to change: Understanding the aides' point of view. *Journal of Long-Term Care Administration, 21*(2), 27–30.

Wellings, C. (1988). Ageist attitudes promote urinary incontinence in older people and can lead to the demoralisation of nursing staff. *Australian Journal on Ageing, 7*(1), 6–15.

Wolf, Z. (1986). Nurses' work: The sacred and the profane. *Holistic Nursing Practice, 1*, 29–35.

Wyman, J., Harkins, S., Choi, S., Taylor, J., & Fantl, A. (1987). Psychological impact of urinary incontinence in women. *Obstetrics and Gynecology, 70*, 378–381.

Yu, L., Johnson, K., Kaltreider, D., Hu, T., Brannon, D., & Ory, M. (1991). Urinary incontinence: Nursing home staff reaction toward residents. *Journal of Gerontological Nursing, 17*(11), 34–41.

Yu, L., & Kaltreider, D. (1987). Stressed nurses dealing with incontinent patients. *Journal of Gerontological Nursing, 13*(1), 27–30.

Yu, L., Kaltreider, D., Hu, T., Igou, J., & Craighead, W. (1989) The ISQ-P measuring stress associated with incontinence. *Journal of Gerontological Nursing, 1*(2), 9–15.

CHAPTER

7

Nursing Care of Incontinent Older Adults

To give an organizational framework to the care provided to incontinent older adults, the philosophy of that care must be made explicit. A philosophy of care is a written statement of beliefs held by an organization about the type of care it provides. The philosophy may be as short as several paragraphs or as long as several pages. The issues in any philosophy-of-care statement, regardless of health care setting, include access to care; quality of care; and individuals' rights to dignity, refusal of treatment, and confidentiality.

A philosophy of continence care should acknowledge the right of a continent person to remain continent and an incontinent individual's right to high-quality care delivered in a compassionate manner, directed to restore or maintain as much normal micturition for as long as possible. It also should include the belief in the importance of the provision of care to maintain the quality of life, self-esteem, and physical and social well-being of individuals who are unable to achieve normal micturition. This philosophy should encompass primary prevention strategies as well as rehabilitative and management strategies.

A philosophy of continence care should also express the importance of continuing education for the staff, older adult, family, and other caregivers, incorporating new information into care as it becomes available. The philosophy of continence care should acknowledge the importance of the establishment of goals compatible with the older adult and caregivers before care is provided. The philosophy should encourage hope for progress, and not promote a sense of hopelessness and futility about treatment.

The type and nature of nursing care stem from the philosophy. For example, because primary prevention strategies are incorporated into a continence care philosophy, nursing interventions are directed toward both continent and incontinent people. Some primary prevention strategies that evolve from a continence philosophy include educating continent adults about perineal care, signs and symptoms of vaginitis and urinary tract infections, weight management, avoidance of fluids with diuretic effects, and pelvic muscle exercises to increase and maintain the tone of the pelvic muscle (Palmer, 1994).

The advances in the understanding of normal micturition, pathophysiology of incontinence, and assessment techniques have led to the development of standards of care for incontinence by professional nursing organizations, e.g., by Wound, Ostomy and Continence Nursing in 1992. Nursing diagnoses developed for continence care include, but are not limited to, altered patterns of urinary elimination, knowledge deficits about bladder-management programs, diversionary activity deficit, potential or impaired skin integrity, ineffective individual coping, ineffective family coping, and toileting self-care deficit (Dittmar, 1989). In order to provide superior effective care, nurses must stay abreast of research advances and new knowledge regarding the care of incontinent adults.

The nursing care of incontinent older adults encompasses information from all the chapters in this book. These chapters should be read prior to or in conjunction with this chapter. Knowledge of causes of incontinence and its associated factors, assessment techniques, and treatment options are essential to providing appropriate and effective care.

The purpose of this chapter is to provide nurses and other members of the nursing staff in all care settings a guideline for providing nursing care to incontinent older adults. Primary prevention, rehabilitation, and strategies to maintain continence are discussed. A "how to" section on establishing a continence program is provided. Readers, however, are encouraged to contact professional medical, nursing, and other organizations to receive updated information about standards of care and research advances. The addresses of several organizations are listed in Appendix B. Rehabilitation of younger individuals who experience altered urinary elimination due to trauma is not addressed, and the reader is referred to rehabilitation nursing textbooks. Sample care plans are provided in this chapter to serve as an illustration of care plans using client and nursing objectives.

The nursing care of incontinent older adults should focus on their cognitive, psychological, and physical needs. The foundation of an effective care plan is the nursing assessment and the information gathered by other members of the health care team. Whenever possible, the older adult should participate in the care planning process. The general goals for restoring bladder function are outlined in Exhibit 7–1. Accurate problem identification is important for the development of realistic, individualized care plans. The care plan should be updated or modified at regular intervals, whenever the status of the older adult changes, and when new information becomes available that affects care.

Exhibit 7–1 Rehabilitation Goals

- To achieve a low amount or no residual urine with adequate emptying of the bladder at predictable intervals
- To prevent complications and preserve renal function
- To maintain skin integrity
- To promote a catheter-free state involving the least amount of time, money, and assistance of other persons
- To establish a bladder program that can be maintained with little interference in social role performance after discharge
- To maintain the client's self-esteem and dignity
- To educate the client and family about
  1. Medications and equipment prescribed when applicable
  2. Prevention and recognition of complications
  3. Performance of the bladder management program
- To assist the client in making any necessary modifications to the home to ensure appropriate toileting facilities
- To obtain maximum client and family participation in and responsibility for the bladder management program

Source: Reprinted from *Rehabilitation Nursing: Process and Application* by S. Dittmar, p. 174, with permission of Mosby-Year Book, © 1989.

NURSING ROLE IN THE CARE OF INCONTINENT OLDER ADULTS

Nurses play a central role in the care of incontinent older adults. In the long-term care, acute care, and home care setting, the nurse may be the only health care professional who detects and begins the assessment and treatment of incontinence. In institutional settings, in addition to providing direct patient care, nurses often write the philosophy of care, standards of care, and policies, and evaluate the job performance of others on the nursing staff. Nurses play the predominant role in defining the mission of the long-term care (Kruzich, 1995). The nurse must function as a change agent, role model to the nursing and other health team members, manager of nursing services, and clinician.

Educator

The nurse functions as an educator to the nursing staff, the affected older adult, family members, and other caregivers. Many people are unaware of normal aging changes, often mistakenly believing that incontinence is a direct consequence of age. During education about continence, the nurse should assess the level of knowledge and provide a brief overview of normal aging changes if needed (see Exhibit 7–2). Affected older adults and families also need to have a basic understanding of the normal structure and function of the urinary tract and the pathophysiology of urinary incontinence. Educational information is widely available from professional organizations and government agencies. Using a model of the urogenital structures, especially when educating women, can facilitate learning of pelvic muscle exercises (Lekan-Rutledge, 1994). The risks and benefits of any intervention should be explained clearly before it is started. The nurse should inform the older adult of the expected intervention outcomes, and explain what the roles of the older adult and staff will be during the intervention. The older adult should also be asked what he or she hopes the intervention will accomplish (Sale & Wyman, 1994). In this way, the nurse and the affected older adult are aware of each other's objectives and expectations of the intervention.

Exhibit 7–2 Normal Aging Changes

Sensory changes
Vision
  Decreased tolerance to glare
  Decreased night vision
  Decreased depth and color perception
  Presbyopia: loss of ability to focus on near objects
Hearing
  Presbycusis: decreased hearing acuity, especially of high frequencies
Taste
  Decreased number of taste buds
  Increased threshold of sensitivity
  Blunted thirst sensation
Olfaction
  Decreased olfaction sensitivity
Touch
  Increased threshold for tactile sensation
Functional changes
  Limited cardiac reserve
  Reduced cough efficiency
  Flexion of hips
  Shift in the center of gravity
  Loss of muscle tone, mass
  Increased reaction time, decreased reflex responses

There are few experts prepared to teach about continence in the nursing school curriculum. Only approximately 2 hours is devoted to classroom teaching about continence (Morishita, Uman, & Pierson, 1994), and ancillary staff members may have received little or no formal continence education in their mandatory certification training. Therefore, in order to educate nurses and the nursing staff effectively, there must be continuing education provided about micturition, effects of age, pathophysiology of incontinence, and available treatment options. By learning to view incontinence as a disruption, the staff can develop nursing strategies that focus on prevention and restoration rather than palliative measures. The staff should receive accurate information about the underlying principles of treatment options, especially regarding the interventions they perform. As discussed in Chapter 5, there are different goals and outcomes for each behavioral therapy. The nursing staff should understand the underlying assumptions about each intervention, the expected outcomes, and the staff's responsibility in providing the intervention.

If the philosophy of continence does not exist or is not conveyed or adopted by the nursing staff, the staff's attitudes and beliefs may adversely affect nursing care. As discussed in Chapter 6, many different attitudes toward urinary incontinence exist. When a nursing staff has an attitude of apathy, hopelessness, or resigned acceptance of incontinence, the attitude can be easily conveyed to the older adult (Wellings, 1988). In turn, the older adult can internalize this attitude, and the incontinent behavior is perpetuated.

The manner in which an episode of transient incontinence is handled is extremely important. A well-meaning attempt to calm and reassure the older adult may be perceived by the older adult as a message that the incontinence is an acceptable or even an expected behavior. The nurse may unwittingly convey the message, "It's OK. We expect incontinence from a person your age." If, after soiled bed linens and clothing are changed, a disposable underpad is placed under the mortified older adult's hips, "just in case," the message is inadvertently reinforced. The staff's expectation that incontinence will occur again can set into motion a variety of behaviors. The staff may start checking and changing the older adult rather than offering toilet access, and the older adult may stop asking to use the toilet, fulfilling the staff's expectations.

When an episode of incontinence occurs, offering words of comfort is important. The nurse should focus on the person's feelings. Statements such as "it must have been embarrassing for this to have happened" and "let's see what we can do so that this won't happen again" are appropriate. The message the nurse sends should be one of empathy and caring, but clearly coupled with an expectation of continence. The focus should be on restoration of continence, rather than incontinence containment.

Clinician

Nurses employ sophisticated interview, physical, psychosocial, and environmental assessment techniques and intervention skills. Nurses obtain in-depth nursing histories; conduct physical, cognitive, and functional assessments; initiate bladder records; develop nursing diagnoses; and work with other health care professionals in the assessment, treatment, and care of incontinent adults. Nurses implement behavioral therapies and evaluate their outcomes. Using available information about the causes and associated factors of incontinence, nurses develop primary prevention interventions in all health care settings. For example, mobility impairments have been associated with incontinence (Jirovec & Wells, 1990). Therefore, mobility enhancement interventions, such as walking and exercise programs, are important components of continence care.

As a clinician, the nurse must assess the effect incontinence has on the psychological well-being and physical health of the individual. Using one of the instruments discussed in Chapter 6 to determine the psychological impact can help the nurse plan activities that will help bolster the individual's self-esteem and ability to cope. Diversionary activities should be planned with occupational therapists and activities personnel to help focus the individual's attention to pleasurable and nonstressful activities.

Skin care is an important component of continence care, especially perineal care for women. Lyder, Clemes-Lowrance, Davis, Sullivan, and Zucker (1992) found that perineal dermatitis can develop within 2 days in older adults with fecal and urine incontinence. Perineal care has its origins in the 19th century in the care of postpartum women (Rhode and Barger, 1990). There is little scientific basis for the frequency and nature of perineal care performed in contemporary nursing practice. However, it has been suggested that perineal care in long-term care should occur each morning, after an incontinent episode, as part of bedtime care, and upon resident request (Warkentin, 1991a). The use of soap and water should be discouraged on aged skin; soap can cause irritation and drying (Klein, 1988). There are many commercially available cleansers. The nurse should carefully select the cleanser best suited to the needs of the incontinent older adult. Saute (1991) outlined elements of the ideal cleanser: "cleans quickly and effectively; neutral or physiologic pH; neutralizes odor; gentle, does not cause burning or stinging; easy to rinse; and contains active antimicrobials" (p. 3).

The nurse also assesses the effects of the environment on the older adult. Location of and access to toilets, ease of removing or adjusting clothing, privacy, and the availability of assistance from staff members are some examples of environmental features the clinician assesses and modifies when appropriate.

Administrator

Many times nurses function in administrative and supervisory roles. Nurse administrators articulate and communicate the philosophy and standard of continence care. Outcome measures are selected and used to determine the effectiveness of interventions. Patient outcomes (such as increased dryness, decreased use of disposable products, and increased self-esteem) may be selected in addition to organizational outcomes (such as decreased laundry costs, high performance during regulatory surveys, and decreased family complaints). Administrators evaluate information about the effectiveness of the care and communicate the findings to the staff. Clearly written expectations for job performance, which includes continence care, and the consequences of superior, adequate, and inadequate job performance must be readily available to staff members. Corrective or remedial administrative actions, which include instituting new policies, modifying policies, and disciplinary actions, are made based on objective, ongoing information obtained for each outcome.

Continence care may require changes in resource allocations. Some changes that may be needed include allocations of funds for the purchase of additional toilet substitutes, commercial cleansers, and external collection devices, and for providing staff members time off and registration fees to attend educational sessions. Job restructuring is another component to continence care. There is evidence that the largest volume of urine loss occurs at night (O'Donnell, Beck & Walls, 1990). Therefore, changes in staffing to ensure sufficient staff to toilet patients at night may be needed.

Researcher

Nursing research provides the scientific basis of nursing care. Many nursing actions are based on tradition rather than on scientific evidence. One example discussed in an earlier section is perineal care. Nurse researchers are actively working to validate current nursing practices as well as identify new techniques of nursing care and those that advance nursing science.

There has been a great deal of nursing research activity investigating the characteristics of incontinent older adults, assessment techniques, and behavioral interventions. Research is necessary to answer questions about the effectiveness of treatment in terms of changing underlying pathophysiology and improving outcomes, for example, decreasing wetness, improving quality of life, and reducing caregiver burden (Wells, 1994). The reader is encouraged to review professional journals, attend local and national educational sessions, and join professional organizations to keep informed about the latest continence research findings.

Nurses, both independently and with others, often conduct research or participate in data collection for a research study investigating questions that arise out of practice. An advantage of being a part of an interprofessional research team is that nurses can pool resources with the other team members, learn from other research perspectives and expertise, and share in a rich database. Participation in the research process provides intellectual stimulation and healthy questioning of current practices. Communication of research findings contributes to the growth of nursing knowledge, to the development of nursing practice, and ultimately to improving the quality of life of affected older adults. Just a few examples of many research issues of interest to nurses are the following:

- Are vaginal weights effective in reducing or preventing incontinence in postmenopausal women?
- What are the effects of the long-term care nursing staff's attitudes and beliefs about urinary incontinence on its compliance with specific behavioral interventions?
- Do specific environmental modifications decrease the prevalence of incontinence in home care clients?
- What effects does bacteriuria have on the frequency of incontinent episodes of long-term care residents?

Through the investigation of care-related questions, nurse researchers can work as partners with clinicians, educators, and administrators to improve continually the treatment and care of incontinent older adults.

NURSING CARE OF INCONTINENT OLDER ADULTS

The sample nursing care plans in this chapter illustrate four types of incontinence or altered urinary elimination frequently found in the older population:

1. Stress urinary incontinence in a postmenopausal woman
2. Altered urinary elimination secondary to prostatic hyperplasia in an older man
3. Transient incontinence secondary to delirium
4. Functional incontinence in a frail, cognitively impaired older woman

A Postmenopausal Woman with Stress Urinary Incontinence

Cognitive Care

The general goal of nursing care for a postmenopausal woman with stress incontinence is to reduce and/or eliminate episodes of urinary leakage with physical exertion. The nurse should provide the older woman information about the normal position and function of the organs comprising the genitourinary tract. The causes of stress urinary incontinence (a sudden increase in pressure within the abdominal cavity and bladder that occurs with a cough or sneeze with abnormal position or movement of the urethra, overwhelming the intraurethral pressure) should be discussed with the older woman. After counseling and educational sessions, the older woman should be able to identify some of her behaviors that may need to be modified or changed to reduce episodes of stress incontinence (e.g., lose weight, stop smoking).

Verbal and written instructions for pelvic muscle exercises should be given to the older woman in terminology appropriate for her individual level of understanding. As a reasonable test for comprehension, the older woman should be able to describe the steps involved in performing pelvic muscle exercises. Before the woman does the pelvic muscle exercises independent of the nurse, the older adult should demonstrate that she has correctly located the pubococcygeus muscle and is able to contract it. The nurse should observe the woman's technique, ensuring that the correct muscle is being contracted by inserting a gloved finger into the woman's vagina, by inserting a periometer into the woman's vagina, or by using biofeedback equipment with surface electrodes applied to the woman's perineum and abdomen. The woman should be instructed to contract the pelvic muscle before she coughs, sneezes, rises from a chair, or performs any physical exertion that causes her to leak urine. Pelvic muscle exercises are described in Chapter 5.

Medications to increase urethral resistance, such as alpha-adrenergics, may be prescribed to treat stress incontinence. The woman should receive complete instructions on the administration of the medication as well as be informed of its side effects. Hormone replacement therapy (e.g., topical estrogen cream) may be used to replenish vaginal and urethral tissues. However, the woman should understand the contraindications and side effects of the cream prior to its administration.

Psychological Care

Urinary incontinence is a condition very distressing to the affected older adult. The nurse should foster a trusting relationship with the older woman by providing a quiet, private environment when taking a history, offering counseling, or giving instructions for care. Use of one of the standardized questionnaires about the effects of incontinence, discussed in Chapter 6, will provide the nurse with important information about the impact of incontinence on lifestyle and the coping techniques the woman uses.

Empathy is essential to the nurse/client relationship. The nurse should always project an attitude of realistic hopefulness. Improvement in pelvic muscle tone is gradual. It may take up to 1 month to notice improvement and up to 3 to 6 months for significant changes (Smith & Newman, 1994). Confidentiality of records and interactions with the client should be strictly maintained.

Promoting self-esteem of the older woman is an integral part of the treatment plan. Encouraging the woman to set realistic goals related to treating urinary incontinence (e.g., "I am going to lose 1½ lb this month" rather than "I am going to lose 25 lb") is an important role of the nurse. Overambitious goals lead to failure, discouragement, and defeat.

The nurse should create an atmosphere that induces the woman to examine her own behaviors and identify acceptable interventions that can be used to modify those behaviors. The nurse should never usurp the woman's independence, be judgmental, or coerce changes in lifestyle not desired by the older woman. Rather, negotiating changes and offering encouragement and support are two paramount nursing actions in providing psychological care to women with stress urinary incontinence. Lasting changes only come about when motivation comes from within.

Physical Care

A woman capable of self-care should be encouraged to resume and/or continue to care for herself. Good personal hygiene measures are important components of physical care. The older woman should be instructed to keep the perineal area clean and dry. Absorbent cotton underwear without tight leg binding may provide more comfort than tight-fitting girdles and nylon underwear. A tight-fitting girdle can push abdominal organs inward and down onto the bladder, resulting in more pressure on the bladder. The older woman should be encouraged to change soiled undergarments and replace moist disposable continence pads, sanitary pads, or panty liners throughout the day. Wearing soiled garments not only is uncomfortable and odor producing, but may increase the risk of skin breakdown and infection in the perineal and vaginal region. Women should be discouraged from douching in their attempt to eliminate odor. Although there is little research on the effects of douching on postmenopausal vaginal tissue, douching may change vaginal pH, eliminate normal vaginal flora, and irritate vaginal tissues. A woman with a heavy or foul-smelling vaginal discharge or bleeding should be referred to a gynecologist. Topical estrogen cream therapy may be needed to relieve symptoms of atrophic vaginitis. Women should be taught to recognize the classic signs and symptoms of urinary tract infections, and to report them to the nurse or physician immediately. Exhibit 7-3 outlines the signs and symptoms of a urinary tract infection.

A weight-reduction program may be another important component in helping the woman to reduce stress episodes. Developing a realistic weight loss program while maintaining adequate nutritional requirements congruent with the older woman's lifestyle may require assistance from a dietician, nutritionist, and/or a physical therapist. The adequate intake of fluid should be discussed. The daily requirement for fluids is 30 ml/kg of body weight (Lipschitz, 1992). Adequate hydration is essential for the woman to experience bladder fullness and for normal micturition to occur. However, the intake of fluids with a diuretic effect, such as caffeinated coffee, tea, and sodas, should be limited.

The woman should be encouraged to empty her bladder when the conscious desire to void is first noticed. She should also be instructed to void in an unhurried manner to facilitate complete emptying. See Sample Care Plan 1 on stress incontinence.

A Man with Benign Prostatic Hyperplasia

Cognitive Care

Explanation of the normal structure, function, and aging of the urinary tract and the prostate gland will help the older man to understand his potential vulnerability

---

Exhibit 7-3 Signs and Symptoms of Urinary Tract Infections

Classic Signs and Symptoms
  Fever or chills
  Flank, lower back, suprapubic pain
  Burning on urination
  Dysuria
  Frequency
  Urgency
  Pyuria
  Microscopic hematuria
Possible Signs and Symptoms
  Delirium or altered mental status
  Decline in ability to perform activities of daily living
  Lethargy
  Decreased appetite

Sample Care Plan 1

Stress Incontinence

Mrs. S is a 69-year-old widow living alone in a high-rise apartment complex for the elderly. She is 5 ft 4 in and weighs 160 lb. During her annual physical examination, Mrs. S told her geriatric nurse practitioner (GNP) that she experiences a small amount of urinary leakage when she coughs, sneezes, or bends over. When questioned, she said that she is unable to stop the flow of urine once it has started. She further stated that she feels extremely embarrassed and is afraid that her friends will discover her problem and ostracize her. She is afraid to travel in other people's cars, fearing that she may soil the seat. Mrs. S is highly motivated to reduce the incontinence and states, "I don't want to get worse!"

Her history reveals that she has mild hypertension. "I'm supposed to lose weight and avoid salt, but I don't do either." She has had no pelvic surgeries, one vaginal delivery 45 years ago, and her last menses was 25 years ago. She takes no prescription medications, but takes a multivitamin tablet daily and occasionally takes a nonprescription sleeping pill. Her bowels move regularly. She gets up once a night, and voids approximately eight times per day.

The physical assessment revealed an obese abdomen with no surgical scars, no signs of vaginitis or inflammation of tissue, and no evidence of organ prolapse. During the vaginal examination with the GNP's gloved finger introitus, Mrs. S was able to contract weakly her pelvic floor muscle. A provocation stress test was positive for leakage. Her bulbocavernosus reflex is intact. She has no hemorrhoids. Her urinalysis and postvoid residual volume were normal.

Nursing Diagnosis:
Alteration in urinary elimination: stress incontinence

Goals:
  Reduce episodes of urinary leakage.
  Improve pelvic muscle strength.

Outcomes:
  1. Mrs. S describes basic etiological factors for stress incontinence.
  2. Mrs. S develops goals for the management of stress incontinence.
  3. Mrs. S demonstrates methods for managing stress incontinence.
  4. Mrs. S remains free of complications related to stress incontinence.

continues

Sample Care Plan 1 continued

Client Objectives:	Nursing Objectives:
Receive help from nurse to stop urinary accidents.	Explain the structure and function of the female genitourinary system. Explain how stress incontinence can occur in women. Instruct Mrs. S to keep bladder record and review it with Mrs. S every 2 weeks.
Perform pelvic muscle exercises.	Give Mrs. S instructions on how to perform pelvic muscle exercises correctly. Provide verbal feedback to ensure compliance. Give portable periometer to assess progress at home.
Decrease odor by changing disposable pads.	Discuss the importance of avoiding constricting undergarments. Promote good personal hygiene. Discourage use of pads as urinary leakage decreases.
Avoid beverages with diuretic effect.	Instruct Mrs. S to avoid beverages with diuretic effect. Give Mrs. S a list of non-caffeinated beverage alternatives.

Goal:
Reduce weight to within range desirable for height and age.

Outcome:
Mrs. S adheres to balanced diet and regular exercise program.

Client Objectives:	Nursing Objectives:
Monitor food intake daily for 1 week.	Review food intake record with Mrs. S for patterns of eating and snacking, and types and amounts of food consumed.
Stop snacking between meals. Stop having dessert seconds. Reduce salt intake.	Record weight on a weekly basis. Provide nutritional information for a balanced reducing diet and for alternatives to salt for seasoning food.

continues

Sample Care Plan 1 continued

State goals for weight reduction of no more than 1 lb per week.	Provide information about principles of safe weight reduction.
Take a walk to tolerance twice a day. Participate in group exercise class twice a week at a local senior center.	Encourage Mrs. S to increase daily exercise gradually through walks and joining an exercise group.

Goal:
Improve self-esteem.

Outcome:
Mrs. S expresses effective coping strategies.

Client Objectives:	Nursing Objectives:
Express concerns to nurse and develop ways of coping with feelings about urinary incontinence.	Empathize with and behave nonjudgmentally toward Mrs. S. Provide psychological support. Help Mrs. S identify sources of support for family and friends. Teach relaxation techniques of imagery and breathing.
Participate in social interactions with friends and family members.	Encourage participation in social activities.
Maintain grooming and physical appearance.	Encourage Mrs. S to wear attractive clothing, hairstyle, and flattering cosmetics. Instruct Mrs. S to avoid scented soaps, powders, and douches. Instruct Mrs. S to wipe the perineum front to back after eliminating.

Nursing Orders:
Request nutritionist consultant.
Weight every month.
Patient education—pelvic muscle exercises, diet, personal hygiene.

to urinary retention and development of overflow incontinence. Most men with prostatic hyperplasia are treated with "watchful waiting," which is the monitoring of symptoms and disease progression by the physician without active interventions (Clinical Practice Guideline Panel, 1994).

Men with mild symptoms should be instructed to limit fluids in the evening and to avoid medications with a urinary retentive effect. Many over-the-counter drugs, especially decongestants, can cause urinary retention. The older man should be instructed to make other health care providers aware that he has benign prostatic hyperplasia and to inform them of *all* medications that he is currently taking.

Psychological Care

The man's urinary tract and prostate gland are inexorably linked to his sexuality and body image. The nurse should be capable of counseling the older man about issues regarding his sexuality. Many fears about aging and death may surface during the counseling sessions. The nurse should feel comfortable about discussing these issues in an open manner and understand that the older man may be reluctant to discuss these issues. If the nurse is uncomfortable or unprepared to deal with these issues, the older man should be referred to another nurse or health care professional prepared to explore the older man's feelings. In making this referral, the nurse should make it clear to the older man that the referral is not a judgment of him, or a rejection of him or his feelings, but is an attempt to give him the best care and advice possible. However, it is within the scope of nursing practice to counsel older adults about sexual issues, and a sexual history should always be a part of the comprehensive health assessment of all older adults.

Physical Care

The nurse should counsel the man to be aware of and regulate the amount of fluid he ingests after dinner to avoid excessive nighttime voidings. Periodic evaluation of the symptoms using the American Urological Association (AUA) symptom index is advisable. See Chapter 4 for evaluation of prostatic hyperplasia.

The bladder should be palpated during a physical examination. An overdistended bladder with a high postvoid residual should be reported to a urologist to prevent an emergency condition of acute retention and to prevent vesicoureteral reflux and renal damage. The older man should be instructed to report immediately to his nurse or physician any of the following: absence of voiding, acute low back pain, and/or abdominal pain.

To facilitate voiding, the older man should have adequate privacy, be in a standing position, and use the technique of manual expression of urine (Credé maneuver). As always, good personal hygiene measures should be encouraged to avoid odor and skin breakdown.

Stasis of urine or high postresidual volumes may increase the likelihood of urinary tract infection. The older man should be alerted to the signs and symptoms of a urinary tract infection (see Exhibit 7–3) and instructed to report any possible signs immediately. Due to changes in the immune system with age, a urinary tract infection may not present with symptoms, especially fever, until it has become far advanced (Cantrell & Norman, 1992).

Prostatic obstruction may be corrected by surgery if pharmacologic (alpha-blockers and finasteride) and other measures (balloon dilation) fail (Clinical Practice Guideline Panel, 1994). See Chapter 5 for a discussion of treatment options. The nurse should understand the underlying principles of each treatment and know the expected outcomes. During and after treatment, the nurse should observe for potential complications, including adverse effects of medications, postoperative complications of perioperative infection, hemorrhage, urinary retention, myocardial infarction, stroke, and incisional complications (Clinical Practice Guideline Panel, 1994). Late complications to surgical interventions include impotence, retrograde ejaculation, incontinence, and urethral stricture (Clinical Practice Guideline Panel, 1994). See Sample Care Plan 2 on prostatic hyperplasia.

An Older Man with Transient Incontinence Secondary to Delirium

In Chapter 3, delirium was identified as a transient cause of urinary incontinence in some older adults. Delirium can cause the older adult to forget the location of the bathroom, forget to go to the toilet, or forget to communicate the need to go to the toilet to others. It can also cause the older adult to be unable to interpret correctly the sensation of bladder fullness or to inhibit voiding.

The most effective treatment of delirium is prevention. Delirium can be caused by pain, infection, additions or changes in medications, sleep disruptions, fluid and electrolyte imbalances, and changes in environment. Individuals with dementia may become delirious, worsening their already impaired cognitive status. It is important that the nurse differentiate between delirium and irreversible cognitive impairments in order to provide nursing interventions that alleviate the delirium by reversing the physiological disruptions and/or modifying the environment to reduce sensory stimulation. A hallmark characteristic of delirium is its sudden onset. Sudden impairment or changes in mobility, vision, and hearing can place an older adult at risk for becoming confused and disoriented. The acronym FANCAPES (fluids, aeration, nutrition, communication, activity, pain, elimination, and socialization) can help the nurse assess for changes in essential human needs that may lead to acute confusional states (Ebersole & Hess, 1994). See Exhibit 7–4.

Sample Care Plan 2

Prostatic Hyperplasia

Mr. J is 78 years old and resides with his wife in their home of 34 years. His wife has been confined to bed for the last 5 years because of a cerebrovascular accident. Mr. J provides most of his wife's nursing care. While the community health nurse was visiting one day, Mr. J mentioned that he was having changes in his voiding habits. He stated that he has a feeling of fullness after voiding, difficulty in initiating urination, dribbling of urine, and getting up several times a night to void. Mr. J stated, "My doctor said that my prostate gland is enlarged and I need an operation. Well, I'm not going to have it. Who would take care of Gladys while I'm in the hospital?" Mr. J, on advice of the nurse, made an appointment with a university-affiliated urology clinic.

Nursing Diagnosis:
Alteration in urinary elimination related to prostatic hyperplasia

Goal:
Promote bladder emptying and prevent urinary retention and overflow incontinence.

Outcomes:
Mr. J will describe basic etiological factors of prostate hyperplasia.
Mr. J and his nurse will develop goals for the management of his prostatic hyperplasia.
Mr. J will demonstrate methods for managing his prostatic hyperplasia.
Mr. J will remain free of complications related to his prostatic hyperplasia.

Client Objectives:	Nursing Objectives:
Avoid waking to void.	Ingest fluids during the day, but restrict fluids after dinner. Obtain history and perform physical exam. Monitor intake and output for fluid imbalance.

continues

Sample Care Plan 2 continued

	Instruct Mr. J to notify physician immediately if voiding in small amounts or if voiding is absent. Administer AUA symptom index and share results with urologist.
Recognize and avoid medications with urinary retentive effects.	Test Mr. J's awareness of medications (including over-the-counter medication) with urinary retentive effects.
Discuss treatment options to relieve outlet obstruction.	Explain various treatment options. Request urologist consult. Instruct Mr. J about positioning to empty bladder, Credé maneuver.
Maintain personal hygiene.	Observe for signs of poor or inadequate hygiene and provide information about personal hygiene.

Goal:
Avoid developing a urinary tract infection.

Outcome:
Urinalysis and urine culture will be negative for bacterial growth.

Client Objectives:	Nursing Objectives:
Recognize the signs and symptoms of urinary tract infection.	Discuss and explain the signs and symptoms of urinary tract infection. Perform microscopic examination of urine. Observe the appearance of urine; do a dipstick test for nitrates and leukocyte esterase.

Goal:
Increase knowledge regarding the changes in the male genitourinary tract.

Outcome:
Mr. J will describe changes in voiding due to prostatic hyperplasia and steps to take to avoid urinary retention.

continues

Sample Care Plan 2 continued

Client Objectives:	Nursing Objectives:
Gain information about aging and sexuality and discuss feelings about aging and sexuality with the nurse.	Provide Mr. J with factual information about aging and sexuality. Provide Mr. J with a private, nonjudgmental forum for discussion.

Nursing Orders:
  Obtain MD/urologist consult.
  Do dipstick test and microscopic examination of urine.
  Monitor fluid intake and output.
  Teach patient about structure and function of male genitourinary tract, medication contraindications, treatment options, sexuality, and aging.

Exhibit 7-4 Assessment of Delirium

Fluids	What is the older adult's level of hydration? Is alcohol withdrawal a factor?
Aeration	Are respiration and aeration of tissues adequate for the older adult's functional level?
Nutrition	Are there any changes or deficits in the older adult's nutritional status? What is the status of the oral cavity?
Communication	How well can the older adult communicate his or her needs?
Activity	Are there changes in the older adult's functional level and ability to participate in activities, including activities of daily living?
Pain	Is the older adult in pain? Are the pain management strategies sufficient?
Elimination	Are there any changes in the older adult's bowel and bladder habits and patterns of elimination?
Socialization and social skills	How well does the older adult function in the company of others? Does the older adult have an opportunity to interact with others?

By correctly identifying the etiology of delirium and taking the necessary corrective actions, the nurse often finds that previously continent older adults regain their bladder control. Generally, as the older adult's sensorium clears, the older adult's previous pattern of continent urinary elimination returns, provided that toilet facilities are available, the person's level of mobility permits access, or assistance is available for using the toilet or toilet substitute.

Cognitive Care

Nursing actions must be intensive when an individual has serious cognitive impairments. Provisions for the older adult's safety are paramount, especially if the older adult is able to be ambulatory.

The nurse should eliminate extraneous noises and lighting that can overload an already disrupted sensorium. When talking with the older adult, the nurse should use a clear, slow voice and speak in short, simple sentences.

Efforts to reorient the confused older adult can be aided by placing in the older adult's living space a clock, a calendar, and familiar personal belongings. Caregivers should wear a name tag with the name printed in large block letters, and the older adult should also be verbally reminded of the caregiver's name on a regular basis.

The use of physical and chemical restraints should be avoided. Confusion and disorientation can be heightened through injudicious use of restraints. The safety and restoration of the cognitive state of the individual should be the top priority of the nurse and all other caregivers. Restraints can be avoided by providing a sitter, using diversionary activities, maximizing the older adult's senses by providing clean and properly fitting eyeglasses and hearing aids, and encouraging the family to visit.

Psychological Care

Losing one's cognitive abilities, even on a temporary basis, is a terrifying experience. The perceived loss of control can lead to panic and increased anxiety. A quiet, reassuring approach by the nurse can help allay some of the anxiety. Allowing and promoting independence in any aspect of care (e.g., feeding oneself) project an unspoken expectation for the older adult to regain control over other aspects of daily living. Praise for maintaining continence must be expressed to the individual through both the verbal and nonverbal actions of the nurse. Consistency in the environment is most important while the pathophysiologic cause of the delirium is being treated. It may be helpful to have the same staff members provide daily care.

The self-esteem of the individual can be bolstered by the nurse in numerous ways, such as listening to the older adult, fixing his or her hair, or taking him or her for a walk. By providing a calm, steady hand to guide the older adult through the frightening experience of sudden cognitive loss, the nurse can alleviate much emotional suffering.

The nurse should use other resources to provide psychological support to the delirious older adult. Family members can give great support to the older adult by sitting quietly by the bedside, assisting in activities of daily living, and reassuring the older adult of continued love and concern. It can be very traumatic for a family member to see the older adult in a confused state. The nurse should be prepared for strong emotional reactions from some family members. Explaining the cause or probable cause of the delirium and the remedial steps being taken by the health professionals can help to alleviate the family's anxiety. The nurse should encourage the family members to promote the independence of the older adult within the realm of safety while not placing excessive demands for immediate restoration of "normal" functioning. The older adult and family members require the calm presence of the nurse to help ease tension and fear.

Physical Care

The scope of physical care for the confused older adult is largely dependent on the cause of the delirium and other medical conditions. If the older adult is frail and debilitated from disease, nursing actions will be intensive. The nurse not only will offer toilet facilities but also will assist the older adult in proper positioning and personal hygiene.

Ideally, a woman should be seated on the commode and a man should stand in front of a commode to provide a strong environmental cue to void. Assistance in removing or replacing clothes and help with personal hygiene should be offered. Incontinent women should be helped to wipe the perineum in a front-to-back motion with toilet tissue to prevent odor and excoriation. Sometimes cleansing the perineal area with a mild commercial cleanser, especially after fecal soiling, is required. Hot water should never be applied to the perineum. The older adult should wash his or her hands after every toileting. The motto "less is better, none is best" should be followed when applying powder to the pubic area. Powder should never be applied directly to the urethral or vaginal openings or in skin folds. If used, any powder or ointments should be applied in a thin layer and all excess wiped away.

The objective of the physical care is to deliver private, sanitary, and effective toileting, while avoiding incontinent episodes. Underlying this objective is the goal of restoring the cognitive functioning, independence, and self-esteem of the older adult. Suggestions for the care of the older adult with transient incontinence secondary to delirium can be found in Sample Care Plan 3.

Sample Care Plan 3

Transient Incontinence Secondary to Delirium

Mr. O is a 77-year-old man admitted in the early evening to the cardiac care unit of a 500-bed hospital after experiencing chest pains at home. During his first in-patient night his nurse reported to the nursing supervisor that Mr. O was found standing in the hall at 2:30 a.m., bleeding from the site of a displaced IV drip, with cardiac monitor leads detached, incontinent of urine, and disoriented to time and place.

Nursing Diagnosis:
Altered urinary pattern secondary to delirium

Goals:
Improve cognitive function.
Restore physiological status.

Outcomes:
Mr. O's caregivers will describe the basic etiological factors of transient incontinence secondary to delirium.
Mr. O's caregivers will develop the goals for a bladder program for Mr. O.
Mr. O's caregivers will provide consistent access to toilet substitutes until Mr. O can resume self-care.
Mr. O will remain free of complications associated with transient incontinence, secondary to delirium (e.g., falls).

Client Objectives:	Nursing Objectives:
Recognize where he is and why.	Monitor cardiac function and blood value; take immediate remedial actions for abnormal values. Ask family member to sit with Mr. O. Reorient Mr. O to his surroundings; explain why he is in the cardiac care unit. Keep call light within reach of patient. Talk to Mr. O in a calm and reassuring voice.

continues

Sample Care Plan 3 continued

	Maximize sensory functioning (proper lighting, glasses, hearing aid, etc.).
	Place familiar photos and personal effects close to Mr. O.
	Avoid restraints.
	Administer back rubs, warm milk to facilitate sleep.
	Orient Mr. O to use of urinal.
	Assist Mr. O with urinal before retiring, on awakening, after meals, and upon his request.
	Keep urinal within Mr. O's reach.
	Assist to stand at bedside to void if condition permits.
	Provide quiet environment to help induce sleep.
	Have clock and calendar in patient room.
	Use heparin lock instead of continuous IV drip and hydrate orally.

Goal:
Avoid injury and facilitate recovery.

Outcome:
Mr. O's hospitalization course will be free of falls, skin tears, and accidental ingestion of harmful substances.

Client Objectives:	Nursing Objectives:
Return home without injury.	Ask family member to stay with Mr. O when condition permits.
	Assist Mr. O to the bathroom.
	Give Mr. O the call light and instructions for use.
	Check patient in person frequently.
	Orientation to time, place, and person.
	Remove swallowable and harmful objects from bedside.

continues

Sample Care Plan 3 continued

	Remove unnecessary clutter and furniture from the room. Assist Mr. O in ambulation when condition permits. Monitor environment for potential danger and modify as needed.

Nursing Orders:
  Assign consistent staff member to Mr. O's care.
  Provide scheduled toileting.
  Monitor cognitive status.
  Monitor physiological status.
  Maintain voiding record.

An Older Adult with Functional Incontinence Secondary to Dementia

The most frequent types of dementia in older adults are Alzheimer's disease and vascular dementia, which includes multi-infarct dementia (Skoog, Nilsson, Palmertz, Arne Andreasson, & Svanborg, 1993). In both types, short-term memory is affected (see Table 7–1).

Although cognitive impairments are prevalent in the older population, dementia is not a result of normal aging. Health care professionals, especially nurses, should actively investigate the causes of the decline in the cognitive status of an older adult and take action to reverse the process or, with dementia, promote the maximal level of functioning.

Dementia is a factor associated with urinary incontinence. That is, many incontinent older adults are cognitively impaired. However, not all cognitively impaired older adults are incontinent. Therefore, the nurse and the entire nursing staff must be motivated by a philosophy of compassionate care that promotes continence and the quality of life by giving assistance in carrying out activities of daily living. This care not only includes providing assistance to achieve regular toileting but also includes the promotion of grooming, helping the person with physical appearance, and making clothing as attractive as possible.

Cognitively impaired older adults can be surprisingly sensitive to nonverbal behaviors. Therefore, the nurse must be aware of unintentional messages sent to the impaired older adult by the nursing staff. For example, if the only time the older adult is touched and receives attention is during the changing of soiled clothing,

Table 7-1 Characteristics of Alzheimer's Disease and Multi-Infarct Dementia

Characteristics	Alzheimer's Disease	Multi-Infarct Dementia
Onset	Gradual	Abrupt
Course	Progressive	Stepwise
Predisposing factors	Down's syndrome	Arterial hypertension
Gender	Slightly more frequent in women	More frequent in men
Progression	Unrelenting	May be halted with early treatment of hypertension and vascular disease
Biology	Theories include Genetic factor Slow-acting virus Autoimmune reaction	History of hypertension, vascular disease, stroke
Physical impairment	Little until advanced stages	May have impairment on one side of the body
Treatment	Symptom management	Vasodilators may help

then unintentionally the incontinent behavior is positively reinforced by the nursing staff. Therefore, techniques of behavioral modification should be incorporated into the nursing care plan. This means that positive behaviors such as remaining continent until the next opportunity to toilet and even making attempts to go to the toilet should be rewarded, both verbally and nonverbally.

Cognitive Care

The level of cognitive impairment varies from forgetfulness and lack of judgment to total inability to communicate needs and to respond to stimulus from the environment and others.

Many times, cognitively impaired older adults are able to communicate verbally the need to void, and ambulatory cognitively impaired individuals can maintain their continence independently or with regular reminders to use the toilet.

Urinary incontinence occurs when older adults are unable to remember the location of the bathroom, unable to remember how to handle buttons and zippers, and even unable to remember a recent urge to void. The environment should have visual cues to remind the older adult to go to the bathroom. Arrows, bright signs, and even footprints painted on the floor leading the way to the toilet facilities are helpful aids in reminding the older adult where and when to go to the bathroom. Using contrasting colors on bathroom doors or applying brightly colored designs on the door can make bathrooms easier to identify (Ouslander & Marks, 1990).

The overall nursing goal is to promote and maintain the level of functioning of the older adult. The nurse and nursing staff must clearly understand the etiology and progression of the cognitive impairment. As the older adult's cognitive status gradually deteriorates, highly developed assessment skills must be employed. The cause of sudden worsening of urinary incontinence must be vigorously investigated. A cognitively impaired older adult has the same potential for developing urinary tract infections, diabetes mellitus, and other causes of transient urinary incontinence as other older adults. The nurse should never assume that a sudden decline in continence status is the result of chronic cognitive impairment.

Psychological Care

Many cognitively impaired older adults suffer from concomitant depression, and urinary incontinence is likely to occur because continence is of low priority for them (Fowler, Ouslander, & Papen, 1990). The amount of energy needed to toilet and maintain one's personal hygiene properly may exceed the amount of energy the individual has to expend. The nurse must have the capacity to relate empathy and concern to the cognitively impaired older adult through verbal and nonverbal communication. Establishing a trusting relationship is vital to providing the individual with the succor needed.

The nurse should be constantly alert for signs of depression in a cognitively impaired older adult. There are effective treatments for depression. When treatment is effective, the quality of life should improve even though the underlying cognitive impairment remains. Therefore, prompt detection and advocation for prompt treatment is necessary.

Establishing a consistent and unhurried routine assists the individual in meeting environmental demands. Familiar objects such as a favorite comb and brush, pictures, family photographs, and even furniture from home can help the individual in an institution to adapt to new surroundings.

The psychological care of the incontinent patient with Alzheimer's disease requires patience, empathy, and the desire on the part of the nursing staff to maintain a human bond with the patient. Good communication and observation skills are essential. A cognitively impaired older adult may express personal needs through channels other than speech. Wandering and pacing may be an attempt to reduce feelings of anxiety and stress. Fidgeting with clothing and general restlessness may be an indication of the need to void. The nurse must have the motivation and the skill to interpret these behaviors and to provide timely assistance to the toilet.

Physical Care

As with delirium, the necessary nursing actions may be varied. Attention must be paid to the personal safety of the older adult. Also, special care must be given to maintaining an adequate fluid intake and activity level. Encouraging personal grooming activities and attention to physical appearance helps the older adult maintain a positive sense of self. The nurse should remember that, due to severe deficits in short-term memory, instructions for activities of daily living must be repeated slowly and simply each time the task is performed.

The nurse should keep a record of the older adult's daily bowel movements. Fecal impaction and urinary tract infections can worsen the incontinence. Maintenance of an oral intake sufficient to meet daily water requirements, regular physical exercises, and providing fiber in the diet promote regular bowel movements and decrease the risk of fecal impaction. The nurse should be knowledgeable about the medications the older adult is taking. Some medications decrease gastrointestinal motility. The physical appearance of urine should be observed. Cloudy, dark, or foul-smelling urine may be indicative of a urinary tract infection. Recent instrumentation of the urinary tract, such as an insertion of a straight or indwelling catheter, can put the older adult at risk of a urinary tract infection. If the older adult exhibits excessive rubbing or scratching of the genital area or wincing or moaning while voiding, an infection may be indicated. See Sample Care Plan 4 on functional incontinence secondary to dementia.

A sudden worsening of cognitive functioning should be assessed thoroughly (see Exhibit 7–4). A cognitively impaired older adult is susceptible to delirium just like other older adults, and the cause must be identified promptly. As physiological factors are assessed, environmental influences must also be explored. The following questions should be asked as the nurse explores for the etiology of the delirium:

- Is the person in pain or acute distress?
- Is an upper respiratory infection or urinary tract infection present?
- What is the fluid and electrolyte status?
- Has the older adult recently experienced a fall or head trauma?
- Is there a change in the serum glucose?
- Is there evidence of fecal impaction or urinary retention?
- Has any concomitant medical condition changed?
- Has there been a change in medications? This includes increases and decreases in dose, additions and deletions of medications, and methods and times of administration.
- Has there been a change in the sleep-wake pattern of the older adult?

Sample Care Plan 4

Functional Incontinence Secondary to Dementia

Mrs. K is an 82-year-old woman with Alzheimer's disease. She has been a resident of a long-term care facility for 2 years. She is very forgetful but responds to simple questions and instructions. Although pleased that Mrs. K is able to dress herself in the morning and ambulates independently but with difficulty, the staff expresses frustration over Mrs. K's inability to remain continent beyond midday. Mrs. K denies that she is incontinent, stating that someone poured water on the floor.

Mrs. K voids eight times a day, six of which are incontinent episodes. Mrs. K cooperates with toileting and enjoys being praised by the staff for looking attractive. Mrs. K is incontinent throughout the day and night. She is continent when a staff member takes her to the bathroom after breakfast. She is continent of stool.

Using the Resident Assessment Profile, the nurse ruled out urological causes of incontinence.

Nursing Diagnosis:
Alteration in urinary elimination: functional incontinence

Goal:
Increase dryness, achieving partial or dependent continence.

Outcomes:
Mrs. K's caregivers will describe the basic etiological factors of functional incontinence.
Mrs. K's caregivers will develop goals for a bladder-management program.
Mrs. K's caregivers will demonstrate appropriate methods for managing functional incontinence.
Mrs. K's caregivers will keep her free of complications related to her functional incontinence.

continues

Sample Care Plan 4 continued

Client Objectives:	Nursing Objectives:
Drink at least 1,200 ml to 1,500 ml of fluid per day.	Monitor fluid intake. Encourage fluids by offering a variety of beverages throughout the day, avoiding caffeinated beverages.
Walk to the bathroom with staff member at least eight times a day.	Observe voiding pattern for at least 3 days; plan prompted voiding according to pattern. Watch for nonverbal cues for signs of need to void. Record Mrs. K's bowel movements. Avoid constipation by physical exercise such as daily walks and group exercise class, fiber in diet, regular time for toileting, and privacy. Prompt Mrs. K to go to the bathroom on awakening, after meals, and before bedtime. Assist when necessary. Praise Mrs. K when she is continent and/or makes attempts to toilet herself. Place identifying signs on door of bathroom. Supply bathroom with toilet paper, adequate lighting, privacy, and clean facilities. Use a calm, reassuring voice when talking to Mrs. K. Assist Mrs. K with eyeglasses, hearing aid, dentures. Assist Mrs. K to dress in attractive, loose clothing with simple fasteners.

Nursing Orders:
  Maintain prompted voiding schedule.
  Assign a regular staff member to Mrs. K.
  Monitor fluid intake and urinary output.
  Keep a record of bowel movements.
  Provide psychological support in an unhurried and reassuring manner.

- Is the individual anemic?
- Are there signs of depression?
- Has the older adult been moved to a new room or a new unit, or been assigned a new roommate?
- Has the caregiver been changed? This can be due to caregiver absence due to illness, vacation, shift rotation, official assignment changes, or informal workload sharing changes among staff members.
- Are the bathroom facilities well lit? Warm? Clean? Is there enough privacy? Enough toilet paper, soap, washcloths, and towels?
- Is the older adult wearing familiar clothing? New clothing? Clothing with difficult and unfamiliar openings?
- Has the environment on the nursing unit been changed in any way? This includes construction, renovation, redecoration, and painting.

The nurse must be able to assess physiological and environmental changes quickly, observe their effect, and be prepared to take remedial action.

The care plan for each cognitively impaired older adult must be tailored to individual needs. As the cognitive impairment evolves, so do the normal physiological changes of aging. The care plan must also take into account the changes that occur from aging on the older adult's ability to function (see Exhibit 7–1). Dementia accompanied by other medical conditions and diseases makes nursing care complex and challenging. Setting realistic goals to be followed consistently by the entire nursing staff leads to effective nursing care of the incontinent, cognitively impaired older adult.

HOW TO SET UP A CONTINENCE PROGRAM

Long-term care facilities in the United States are mandated to improve or maintain as much normal bladder function as possible (Department of Health and Human Services, 1989). Nursing measures to restore and rehabilitate bladder function now take the place of containment and management measures. The focus has shifted from incontinence care to the provision of continence care.

This section discusses factors that facilitate or hinder the establishment and maintenance of continence programs. Exhibit 7–5 lists the antecedents needed to establish a continence program. As with any major program that involves changing behavior, continence programs require diligent planning, realistic outcome measures, strategies to overcome resistance to change, and consistent surveillance to monitor the program's effectiveness. Continence programs may be limited, offering one type of behavioral therapy to a select group of affected adults or they

Exhibit 7–5 Antecedents to Implementation of a Continence Program

Antecedent	Rationale
Philosophy of continence care	The belief that a maximal level of continence is achievable guides nursing actions. Array of interventions includes prevention of incontinence, restoration, and rehabilitation, as well as management strategies. The written statement attests to the belief that continence is expected and possible, and that continence programs are part of the standard of care.
Administrative support	Valuation of continence must be evident at all levels of the organization. Administrative support includes development of policies, job descriptions, performance evaluations, provision of resources such as equipment and supplies, and ongoing education for staff, older adults, and family. Administration must articulate its expectations for the continence programs in terms of desired outcomes and individual accountability.
Education of staff, older adults, and families	Information is a necessary component of behavioral therapies. Adults need explanations and rationales to change behavior. People should receive at least a basic-level explanation of normal micturition, the effects of age, the causes of incontinence, and the principles underlying the different behavioral therapies. Expectations for each therapy should be addressed as well.
Resources	Additional resources will be necessary as assessment and treatment of incontinence take place. These resources may include an examination room and equipment, a selection of external collection devices, automated bladder records, and data management capability.
Collaboration with other disciplines	Physicians, social workers, physical therapists, occupational therapists, activities personnel, and housekeeping staff are some of the other disciplines affected by incontinent older adults. Enlisting their support in the planning stages of continence programs is vitally important to receiving their assistance in assessing incontinence and receiving their cooperation with behavioral therapies that involve consistent, regular toileting.

continues

Exhibit 7–5 continued

Antecedent	Rationale
Environmental modifications	Easy access to toilets is essential. Addition of toilets, toilet substitutes, and urinals may be necessary. Signs, support railings, and nonslip floor strips aid in independent toileting.
Anticipation of resistance to change	Modifying behavior is difficult, and people often resist increased control by others. Including staff input and active participation in planning, enlisting cooperation of key staff members, clearly explaining changes in work patterns, and providing meaningful incentives can help to reduce resistance.

may be comprehensive, incorporating several behavioral interventions, use of supportive devices and equipment, and primary prevention strategies (e.g., teaching continent women pelvic muscle exercises, establishing walking programs to maintain independent access to the toilets). Continence programs vary from facility to facility and reflect the philosophy of continence care of each organization. Some facilities may need to start a continence program on a limited basis, with plans to expand it to include additional interventions in the future. Before any older adult is included in a continence program, a complete assessment must be performed.

Attitudes and Beliefs

The staff's level of knowledge and attitudes toward continence and incontinence in older adults have been identified as important components of continence programs. Many staff members are not aware of the multiple causes of incontinence and believe that incontinence is simply a normal part of aging (Wagner & Colling, 1993; Palmer, 1995). There are reports that some nursing staff members believe incontinence is an attention-seeking behavior (Fonda & Nickless, 1987). The beliefs and attitudes of the nursing staff influence the norms of the work environment. If the geriatric nursing assistant and the first-line manager expect the older adult to be incontinent, and view the assistant's job as one of changing wet clothing, there will be little effort to challenge actual care practices and to provide rehabilitative interventions, regardless of the written philosophy of continence care. The philosophy should be a working document, evident in all standards of care and actual nursing practice.

Many of the beliefs of the nursing staff influence job performance. In one study, despite in-service education, job performance in terms of number of assisted toiletings did not improve (Wagner & Colling, 1993). In another study investigating the effectiveness of prompted voiding, Harke & Richgels (1992) observed that the nursing staff had intervention goals different from those of the research team. The staff expected the intervention to "cure" the incontinence in all of the incontinent residents, resulting in less work for themselves. Therefore, when a continence program is in the planning stages, communication and discussion of the expectations and outcomes of the program must take place. Administrators, clinicians, supervisors, and other caregivers will have different perspectives and expectations. To avoid disappointment and disillusionment in the program, having frank discussions and reaching a consensus about the goals of the continence program are necessary. Individual goals will be developed for each older adult who participates in the program. Because the nursing staff is responsible for carrying out the continence interventions, staff ownership of the program is advised (Harke & Richgels, 1992).

Some individuals may be able to achieve independent continence, while others achieve dependent continence, partial continence, or social continence. The expected outcomes should be stated explicitly prior to the intervention. Periodic evaluation may indicate a need to modify the interventions and expected outcomes for each resident. By knowing and understanding the anticipated outcomes there is no ambiguity about what the staff should expect.

The ancillary nursing staff may resist the administration's control and attempt to exert its own control of the work process (Foner, 1994). Geriatric nursing assistants often feel that the administration overlooks their needs and concerns and creates unnecessary barriers, making the work more difficult and unpleasant (Foner, 1994). These issues must be considered when planning a continence program. A program may look good on paper, but will fail if the staff does not, for whatever reason, carry it out. Therefore, administrative and nursing staff support of the program is essential to its success. Meaningful incentives for the caregivers to carry out the continence interventions must be established and communicated, as well as the consequences of inadequate job performance. The nursing staff's suggestions for implementing or modifying the program must receive serious administrative attention as well. Using the wording suggested by the staff members, soliciting anonymous feedback on questionnaires, and providing support and recognition are suggested components of a successful continence program

(Warkentin, 1991b). Attention to the pride and self-esteem of the staff is another factor that should not be ignored as a continence program is being planned and implemented (Wagner & Colling, 1993). The licensed nursing staff must take a professional interest in the continence program as well, viewing it as a vital component of the standard of nursing care.

Organizational Issues

Some organizational system barriers to continence programs are staffing shortages, inconsistent assignments, and inconsistent supervision. These are administrative issues that must be addressed prior to planning a continence program. There may be a need for shifting workloads and/or job restructuring for geriatric nursing assistants and their immediate supervisors. These issues must be addressed by each facility. Because incontinence affects more than the nursing staff, interdepartmental planning and education should occur. Incontinence affects personnel in laundry, administration, and housekeeping departments. Therefore, continence should be perceived and approached as an organizational issue, rather than solely a nursing issue.

Evaluation

To determine the effectiveness of a continence program, comparisons of specific indicators measured before and after the start of the program are needed. An automated quality control program, described in Chapter 5, involves calculating statistics for each incontinent older adult and monitoring the data for changes indicating improvement or deterioration (Schnelle, 1991; McNees, Stone, Agnew, Schnelle, & Fisher, 1992).

Another method of evaluation includes monitoring staff performance (e.g., the actual number of the expected number of assisted toileting carried out). This number is calculated from forms the geriatric nursing assistant completes after each prompted voiding. To ensure accuracy of the documentation, caregivers responsible for providing prompted voiding or other behavioral interventions are unobtrusively observed at random times during the day to determine whether the intervention is performed. Verbal individual feedback is given to the caregiver on a weekly basis regarding the level of performance (Palmer, Bennett, Marks, McCormick, & Engel, 1994). In another study, 80% or more correctly completed interventions resulted in praise and less than 80% resulted in more attentive supervision (Burgio, Engel, Hawkins, McCormick, & Scheve, 1990).

Continence programs require careful planning. The philosophy and standards of continence care guide the development of the program. The attitudes and beliefs of the nursing staff, older adults, families, and other caregivers must be understood and acknowledged. Myths and misconceptions about incontinence must be nonjudgmentally but firmly and consistently corrected. Development and implementation of administrative policies and allocation of resources appropriate for the scope of the continence program must occur. There are many factors that can hinder the establishment and maintenance of a continence program. Strategies must be developed to nullify or counteract these factors. These barriers include inadequate staffing for the scope of the program; lack of staff participation in the planning of the program; and inadequate resources, including supplies and equipment and time for ongoing in-service education. Other barriers are lack of toilet substitutes; obscure signage to indicate location of toilets; insufficient staff understanding of normal structures and function of the male and female genitourinary tract; the causes of and factors related to incontinence; the treatment options and the rationale for their use; the goals of treatment options; insufficient administrative support resulting in lack of meaningful incentives to the staff to implement the program; lack of sufficient or consistent supervision, including positive feedback as well as remedial counseling; inadequate data management, causing a dearth of information on the effectiveness of the intervention; lack of professional interest in the program by administrators, nurses, and other health care providers; and lack of primary prevention and continence enhancement strategies such as walking and exercise programs, focus on personal hygiene, and handwashing.

Facilities that successfully implement and maintain continence programs enjoy a sense of accomplishment and pride in the care provided (McNees et al., 1992). Careful planning, consistent implementation, and ongoing evaluation are needed for a successful program.

CONCLUSION

The nursing care of incontinent older adults involves many skills. Skills for assessing cognitive, psychological, functional, and physiological status of the individual must be finely tuned and highly developed. The nurse must be able to assess the physical environment for safety hazards; barriers limiting access to the toilet facilities; and the quality, quantity, and location of the toilet facilities. The emotional environment and cultural norms must also come under the nurse's scrutiny. The attitudes and beliefs of the nursing staff, family members, other older adults, and the incontinent older adult must be explored.

Education of the staff, affected older adults, family, and other caregivers is essential. Topics that should be covered include the normal structures and function of the genitourinary tract, the effects of age, and the goals and expectations of different treatment options. This information is necessary for the staff, older adult, and family to develop a realistic outlook toward the care. Nurses need to be armed with sophisticated verbal and nonverbal skills to communicate effectively. Only through an attitude of realistic hopefulness and cooperation by a staff committed to a philosophy of continence and well versed in the nursing care of incontinent older adults will effective, individualized care plans evolve.

The comprehensive assessment and problem identification perspective that nurses have make the nurse the appropriate leader in the development of standards of care for the incontinent older adult. The nurse collects the information needed to plan treatment and makes referrals to other appropriate health care providers. The nursing role in the care of incontinent older adults is multifaceted: educator, clinician, supervisor, and researcher. At times, the nurse is a patient advocate seeking consultations with psychiatrists, social workers, physical therapists, occupational therapists, physicians, and other nurses to improve the quality of life and quality of care.

Because of the rapidly changing health care environment and evolving knowledge and technology, the nurse must stay current regarding the latest research literature and information about new supplies and equipment. Sharing this knowledge with the nursing staff emphasizes the need for skilled and caring nursing personnel to assist older adults to regain control and self-esteem through continence.

REFERENCES

Burgio, L., Engel, B., Hawkins, A., McCormick, K., & Scheve, A. (1990). A staff management system for maintaining improvements in continence in elderly nursing home residents. *Journal of Applied Behavior Analysis, 23*, 111–118.

Cantrell, M., & Norman, D. (1992). Management of common clinical infectious problems. In J. Evans & T.F. Williams (Eds.), *Oxford textbook of geriatric medicine*. New York: Oxford University Press.

Clinical Practice Guideline Panel. (1994). *Clinical practice guideline: Benign prostatic hyperplasia: Diagnosis and treatment* (AHCPR Pub. No. 94-0582). Rockville, MD: Agency for Health Care Policy and Research, Public Health Service, U.S. Department of Health and Human Services.

Department of Health and Human Services. (1989). Rules and regulations: Urinary incontinence. *Federal Register, 54*, 5333–5334.

Dittmar, S. (1989). *Rehabilitation nursing: Process and applications*. St. Louis: Mosby.

Ebersole, P., & Hess, P. (1994). *Toward healthy aging: Human needs and nursing responses* (4th ed.). St. Louis: Mosby.

Fonda, D., & Nickless (1987). Survey of knowledge of staff about urinary incontinence. *Australian Journal on Ageing, 6*, 14–18.

Foner, N. (1994). *The caregiver dilemma.* Berkeley, CA: University of California Press.

Fowler, E., Ouslander, J., & Papen, J. (1990). Managing incontinence in the nursing home population. *Journal of Enterostomal Therapy, 17*, 77–86.

Harke, J., & Richgels, K. (1992). Barriers to implementing a continence program in nursing homes. *Clinical Nursing Research, 1*, 158–168.

Jirovec, M., & Wells, T. (1990). Urinary incontinence in nursing home residents with dementia: The mobility-cognition paradigm. *Applied Nursing Research, 3*, 112–117.

Klein, L. (1988). Maintenance of healthy skin. *Journal of Enterostomal Therapy, 15*, 227–231.

Kruzich, J. (1995). Empowering organizational contexts: Patterns and predictors of perceived decision-making influence among staff in nursing homes. *Gerontologist, 35*, 207–216.

Lekan-Rutledge, D. (1994). Soft sculpture model for teaching pelvic muscle exercise. *Urologic Nursing, 14*, 26–27.

Lipschitz, D. (1992). Nutrition and ageing. In J. Evans & T.F. Williams (Eds.), *Oxford textbook of geriatric medicine.* New York: Oxford University Press.

Lyder, C., Clemes-Lowrance, C., Davis, A., Sullivan, L., & Zucker, A. (1992). Structured skin care regimen to prevent perineal dermatitis in the elderly. *Journal of Enterostomal Therapy, 19*, 12–16.

McNees, M., Stone, S., Agnew, J., Schnelle, J., & Fisher, J. (1992). Alaska nursing home takes national role in addressing urinary incontinence. *Alaska Medicine, 34*, 101–102.

Morishita, L., Uman, G., & Pierson, C. (1994). Education on adult urinary incontinence in nursing school curriculum: Can it be done in two hours? *Nursing Outlook, 42*(3), 123–129.

O'Donnell, P., Beck, C., & Walls, R. (1990). Serial incontinence assessment in elderly inpatient men. *Journal of Rehabilitation Research, 27*, 1–8.

Ouslander, J., & Marks, J. (1990). The management of urinary incontinence in dementia. In N. Mace (Ed.), *Dementia care: Patient, family, and community.* Baltimore: Johns Hopkins Press.

Palmer, M. (1994). A health promotion perspective of urinary continence. *Nursing Outlook, 42*(4), 163–169.

Palmer, M. (1995). Nurses' knowledge and beliefs about continence interventions in long-term care. *Journal of Advanced Nursing, 21*, 1065–1072.

Palmer, M., Bennett, R., Marks, J., McCormick, K., & Engel, B. (1994). Urinary incontinence: A program that works. *Journal of Long-Term Care Administration, 22*(2), 19–25.

Rhode, M., & Barger, M. (1990). Perineal care then and now. *Journal of Nurse-Midwifery, 35*, 220–230.

Sale, P., & Wyman, J. (1994). Achievement of goals associated with bladder training by older incontinent women. *Applied Nursing Research, 7*(2), 93–96.

Saute, R. (1991, December). The evils of soap and water versus medically designed cleansers. *Wound & Skin Care, 1*, 3, 10.

Schnelle, J. (1991). *Managing urinary incontinence in the elderly.* New York: Springer.

Skoog, I., Nilsson, L., Palmertz, B., Arne Andreasson, L., & Svanborg, A. (1993). A population-based study of dementia in 85-year-olds. *New England Journal of Medicine, 328*, 153–158.

Smith, D., & Newman, D. (1994). Basic elements of biofeedback therapy for pelvic muscle rehabilitation. *Urologic Nursing, 14*(3), 130–135.

Wagner, A., & Colling, J. (1993). Resistance to change: Understanding the aides' point of view. *Journal of Long-Term Care Administration, 21*(2), 27–30.

Warkentin, R. (1991a). How frequently should perineal care be done? *Perspectives, 15*(1), 11–13.

Warkentin, R. (1991b). Implementation of a urinary continence program. *Journal of Gerontological Nursing, 18*(1), 31–36.

Wellings, C. (1988). Ageist attitudes promote urinary incontinence in older people and can lead to the demoralisation of nursing staff. *Australian Journal on Ageing, 7*(1), 6–15.

Wells, T. (1994). Nursing research on urinary incontinence. *Urologic Nursing, 14*(3), 109–112.

CHAPTER

8

Supportive Devices for Urine Control

OVERVIEW

Many supportive devices are now available to affected older adults and caregivers to assist and supplement urine control. One purpose of this chapter is to acquaint the reader with some of the products currently on the market and in use. However, no endorsement of any of the individual products presented is intended. Another purpose of this chapter is to assist the reader in identifying the role a device should serve during treatment, and whether the use of a specific product is congruent with treatment goals.

The products discussed in this chapter can be used in different treatment modalities. One product may be used as a primary, permanent treatment, as in social continence, with a goal to keep the individual dry, odor-free, comfortable, and participating in the social environment without embarrassment. Another product may be used only to maintain continence at certain times of the day or under certain conditions, such as during the night or while the person is in bed. Products may also be used as temporary treatment in conjunction with a behavioral intervention. As the person subsequently becomes more dry, the use of a device or product may decrease. However, before any product is used, a thorough assessment of the causes of incontinence must be performed and the goals of treatment clearly stated (see Table 8–1). As always, consideration must be given to the individual's lifestyle, personal preferences, and unique needs. The presence of fecal incontinence and other confounding conditions must also be considered. Products should never be selected with the staff's convenience as the sole justification for use.

The proper equipment can help the incontinent older adult regain independence or at least some measure of control over urinary incontinence, thereby helping to restore dignity and self-esteem. The proper equipment may ease the financial impact that unchecked urinary incontinence entails.

Table 8–1 Congruence Among Behavioral Therapies, Outcomes, and Devices

Behavioral Therapies	Goal	Outcome	Device
Scheduled toileting	Increase dryness and promote quality of life and skin integrity	Partial or dependent continence	Absorbent products; bed protectors; toilet substitutes
Habit training	Use individual's voiding pattern to increase dryness; maintain skin integrity; promote quality of life	Partial or dependent continence	Toilet substitutes; clothing; environmental modifications
Bladder training	Rehabilitate to normal micturition pattern; decrease dependence on products	Independent or dependent continence	Toilet substitutes; dampness detectors
Prompted voiding	Increase staff assistance; increase dryness and awareness of the need to void	Partial or dependent continence	Environmental modifications; clothing; toilet substitutes
Self-management, including pelvic muscle exercise	Decrease leakage and use of absorbent products; promote self-care	Independent or partial continence	Toilet substitutes; environmental modifications; timing devices; absorbent products
Check and change	Contain urine loss and promote quality of life and skin integrity; keep person odor-free	Social continence	External collection devices; absorbent products; clothing; bed protectors; dampness detectors; toilet substitutes

DISPOSABLE ABSORBENT PRODUCTS

A popular product used to contain urine is the disposable adult brief. Some briefs are designed with elasticized legs and have self-adhesive tabs that secure to the brief, ensuring a close fit. These briefs are designed to absorb urine and minimize odor while keeping the skin dry. Since there are several brands available, comparisons of features among the brands should be made to best meet an individual's needs and concerns. Presently there are no industrywide standards regarding absorption, comfort, and capacity.

The most obvious feature is the efficiency of absorption and amount of urinary leakage from the briefs. Briefs should be able to absorb large amounts of urine from a rapid urine flow without leakage. The bulkiness of fit under clothing is another important feature. Besides bulk, some briefs may make noise as the wearer moves, thus revealing the presence of the briefs to others. For the older adult wishing to conceal a problem with the urinary incontinence, bulkiness and noise may make a product unsuitable. Briefs should be assessed for physical comfort because the waterproof material covering the briefs may feel hot and uncomfortable for some wearers. Comfort is an issue, even for people who are unable to give voice to their discomfort. The caregiver must watch carefully changes in behavior such as heightened restlessness, agitation, or picking at the briefs or clothing.

Many older adults have stiff joints and fingers, making ease of changing the briefs a major consideration. Buttons, snaps, and self-adhesive strips can present difficulties to the older adult with impaired manual dexterity. Consideration should also be given to the ease with which the briefs can be changed by wearers who are nonambulatory and by members of the nursing staff.

Other features that must be considered in selecting a particular brand of briefs is protection of the skin against breakdown, the development of urinary tract infections or vaginitis, required changing frequencies, and efficiency of odor control. Effective odor control is essential for an incontinent older adult to maintain social acceptance by others.

The two main advantages of disposable briefs emphasized by the manufacturers are the degree of peace of mind an incontinent older adult experiences when wearing the briefs and the increased physical comfort because wetness against skin is minimized. However, a major concern that must be considered before utilizing briefs is the unspoken but unavoidable conclusion that the individual's incontinence is intractable, and the best that can be achieved is social continence. A potentially treatable incontinence could go untreated, worsen, or go undetected through indiscriminate use of adult briefs. The similarity of disposable briefs to disposable diapers for infants is another concern. The psychological impact on the older adult from the use of the briefs must be carefully assessed. When briefs are selected in the care of an incontinent older adult, the briefs must never be referred to as diapers by the caregivers. The caregiver must not overtly or subconsciously infantilize the older adult who is wearing briefs.

Another type of disposable product is an undergarment that leaves the hip area exposed, thereby reducing some of the bulk. Some are designed with self-adhesive straps that encircle the hips, while others are strapless and rely on special mesh underwear or snugly fitting underwear to hold the underpad in place.

Disposable pads attached to the underwear or panties with an adhesive strip are also widely available. Urine absorption varies among the different brands; therefore careful assessment of the amount and frequency of urine loss, fit, adhesive quality, odor control, comfort, ease of use, and expense are all important considerations. Bierwirth (1992) reported that panty liners and minipads had poor absorption, less than 6 ml; maxipads had slightly larger absorption, approximately 20–70 ml; and adult incontinence pads had the highest absorption, approximately 200 ml. Cottenden (1988) noted that some men are resistant to using pads because of the association with feminine hygiene products. For men with small to moderate amounts of urine loss, there are specially designed urine drip collectors or shields that fit over the penis and either adhere to the underwear or are secured with snugly fitting underwear (Help for Incontinent People, 1994).

REUSABLE BRIEFS AND PRODUCTS

A product similar to the disposable briefs is the disposable pad insert placed in a washable knit brief. The pad is filled with a hydrophilic gel or a cellulose product. The hydrophilic gel is very absorbent. Approximately 1 g of gel absorbs 50 g of urine (Cottenden, 1988).

Reusable briefs with a disposable pad insert or liner are similar to the marsupial pant Willington described in 1969. The pant component was made of knitted polypropylene material with a hydrophobic material next to the skin and a waterproof material on the outside. It was secured at the sides with Velcro. The pad, which slid down into a pouch that fitted over the perineum, had a capacity up to 300 ml of urine. Odor control was considered efficient, allowing social acceptance by others.

Currently, the briefs, made of a blend of nylon and polyester or all cotton, are usually less bulky than the disposable adult briefs (see Figure 8–1). Consequently they may be more comfortable to the ambulant wearer. Standing and looking sharply down to change the pad can compress the carotid arteries, causing lightheadedness and increasing the risk of falling. To change a used pad safely the wearer must be seated and the briefs pulled down. Some pads are flushable, but most are disposed of in the same manner as sanitary napkins.

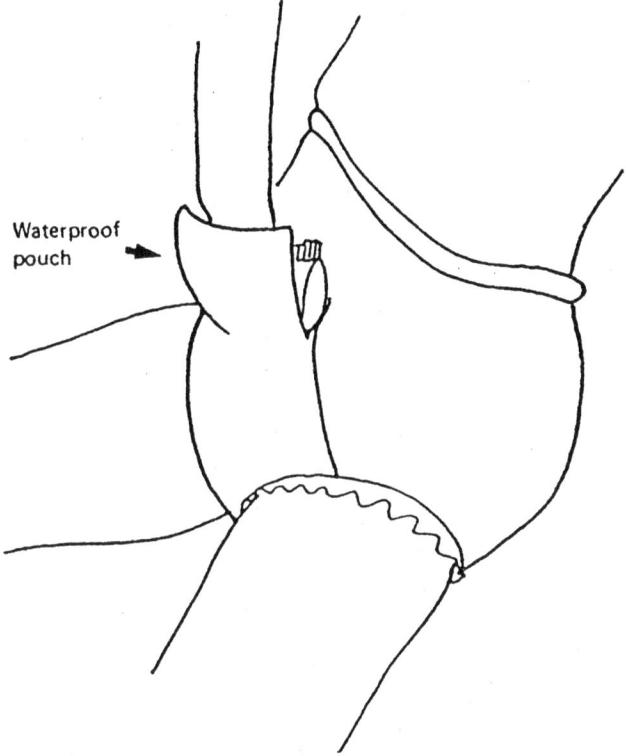

Figure 8–1 Marsupial Pants. *Source:* Reprinted from Smith, N., Aids for Urinary Incontinence, *British Medical Journal*, Vol. 296, p. 772, with permission of the BMJ Publishing Group, © 1988.

Although the knit briefs with the disposable pad are less bulky than the disposable briefs, they may not be suitable for many incontinent older adults. Older adults with limited mobility and manual dexterity may encounter difficulty in changing the pad. A caregiver giving assistance in changing the pad may find it awkward to remove and insert a pad that was designed for wearer handling. Some pads are inserted inside a sleeve or knit webbing of the briefs to keep the pad secure. However, this material will remain in contact with the skin after soiling. In cases of fecal incontinence concomitant with urinary incontinence, the entire system (pad and briefs) should be changed when either type of soiling occurs, and perineal care provided. A secure fit is critical to the prevention of leakage (Clancy & Malone-Lee, 1991). The additional work of laundering the reusable brief needs to be considered when assessing the suitability of a product. Again, the individual needs, economic factors, and expectations of the equipment must be taken into consideration when the older adult and/or caregiver seeks products to provide urine control. The briefs and pads are not meant to substitute for human intervention in providing care to the incontinent older adult. Every attempt should still be made to assist the individual wearing adult briefs or pads to void in the socially appropriate manner using proper toilet facilities.

ABSORBENT BED PROTECTORS

For those individuals with nighttime incontinence, protection of the individual's skin and bed linens is needed. For example, one of the first reusable draw sheets for incontinence is the Kylie sheet, which was first used in Australia. It is composed of two layers. The top layer is porous and water repellent. The inner layer is composed of absorbent material (Pottle, 1986).

The disposable and reusable bed protectors currently available usually have an absorbent layer and a waterproof backing. Large amounts of urine are absorbed while the skin remains dry, thus deterring skin breakdown. Some considerations when selecting bed protectors include skin protection, comfort, amount of urine that can be absorbed, leakage, and whether it will stay in place, especially if the individual is restless (Clancy, 1989). Family caregivers who prefer reusable bed protectors over disposable ones need to ensure that detergents are adequately rinsed from the sheet in order to prevent skin irritation.

ABSORBENT DISPOSABLE BED PROTECTORS

Absorbent disposable pads have been in widespread use in the United States for many years. An absorbent layer of the pad is placed against the individual's skin while an outer waterproof layer protects the bed linens from the urine. Pooling of urine and spillover into bed linens can occur when large amounts of urine are voided.

Absorbent underpads utilizing super-absorbent polymers have been introduced recently to accommodate large amounts of urine and to decrease odor. Proper placement of the pads under the individual is crucial to the success of any underpad protection. Overpadding the bed with multiple pads is costly and unnecessary and should be avoided. Removing wet pads, providing skin care, and frequently repositioning the individual are essential to the health of the individual.

ENVIRONMENTAL MODIFICATIONS

Falling is one of the greatest fears of older adults. If toilet facilities are perceived as unsafe, they will not be used. Stalls too small in which to maneuver, toilets too low, the absence of rails to secure one's balance, the absence of a hook on which to place one's purse or belongings, and lack of privacy are just some of the conditions that make toilet facilities unacceptable and dangerous to the older adult. Grab bars, armrests, and devices that raise the height of the toilet seats, all of which serve to make toilet facilities more accommodating to older adults, are readily available from medical supply stores and catalogues. Application of nonskid strips on the floor in front of the toilet can help the older person to secure footing. Brink & Wells (1986) recommended that the height of the toilet should be between 15 and 20 inches to assist the older adult to rise from the seat.

Of course, limited mobility or difficulty ambulating can make even adequate facilities inaccessible to the individual. Timely access to the toilet is an essential component to the maintenance of continence. Therefore, environmental modifications to ease access and decrease the need for assistance from others are necessary. Toilets, made accessible to the older adult both by features and location, should be clean, well lit, and private but with an efficient call system (see Exhibit 8–1).

Exhibit 8–1 Important Features in the Design of Toilet, Toilet Supplements, and the Environment

Toilets
   Location (i.e., distance)
   Access
      Removal of barriers
      Adequate lighting
      Call system
      Bathroom door design
   Adequate space
      Accommodations of wheelchairs, walkers, and caregivers' help
   Seat height
   Appropriately located grab bars
Commodes
   Adequate number (in institutions)
   Ease and safety of transport
   Design to facilitate support and safety in patient transfer
Bedpans
   Facilitate use in sitting position
   Fracture pan design
Urinals
   Adequate handles
   Curvature to prevent leakage

Source: Reprinted from Brink, C. and Wells, T., Environmental Support for Geriatric Incontinence, *Clinics in Geriatric Medicine*, Vol. 1, No. 4, p. 833, with permission of W. B. Saunders, © 1986.

BEDSIDE COMMODES

Bedside commodes may become necessary for the older adult to regain or retain continence. The commodes come in two types: mobile and stationary. Their designs range in style from utilitarian to the attractive look of bedroom or casual furniture.

Mobile commodes, although convenient for the staff, can present a safety hazard if the older adult attempts to sit while the wheels are unlocked. An over-the-toilet commode, which is an open toilet seat on a movable frame, is another type of mobile commode. The individual is placed on an open seat and wheeled to the toilet. A serious drawback of this type of commode is the inability of some individuals to retain urine while sitting on an open seat. The environmental cue of an open seat to begin urination may be too strong to overcome. Makeshift commodes, such as a bedpan placed on a chair, should never be used as a substitute for a bedside commode, for obvious safety reasons. Every attempt should be made to obtain a bedside commode, and adequate numbers of bedside commodes should be available in the institutional setting. Privacy, toilet paper, and a means for washing the hands should always be available to the older adult who is using a permanent bedside commode. If bedside commodes are shared among patients, the institutional infection control policy for cleaning and disinfecting them must be strictly enforced. A commercially available prepared liquid to control odors may be used in conjunction with, not as a substitute for, regular cleaning.

URINALS FOR MEN

Urinals for men have been in use for centuries. Figure 8–2 illustrates a fairly typical design for a urinal for men. The neck should be wide enough for easy handling. Standing and sitting are the preferred positions for men to use a urinal, especially for men with prostatic hyperplasia and/or mild urinary obstruction. A man who must stand to void but who is unsteady on his feet or unable to hold the urinal will require assistance from the caregiver. There are some urinals designed to prevent leaks and spills if dropped or placed in a nonupright position.

URINALS FOR WOMEN

Urinals for women are commercial available, although not in widespread use (see Figure 8–3). A woman with limited abduction of the hips and thighs would likely find a female urinal uncomfortable to use. Female urinals vary slightly in design. Usually they have a wide opening to encircle the labia and perineum.

Supportive Devices for Urine Control 169

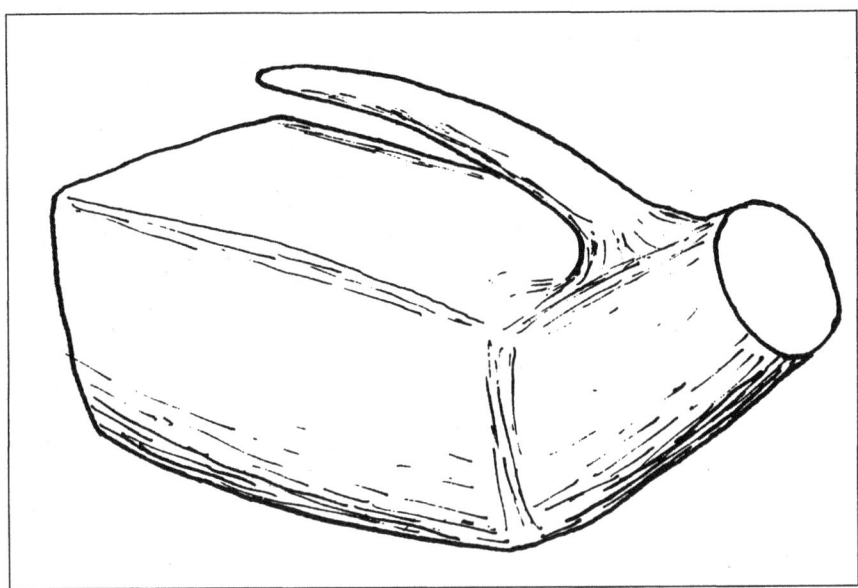

Figure 8–2 Urinal for Men

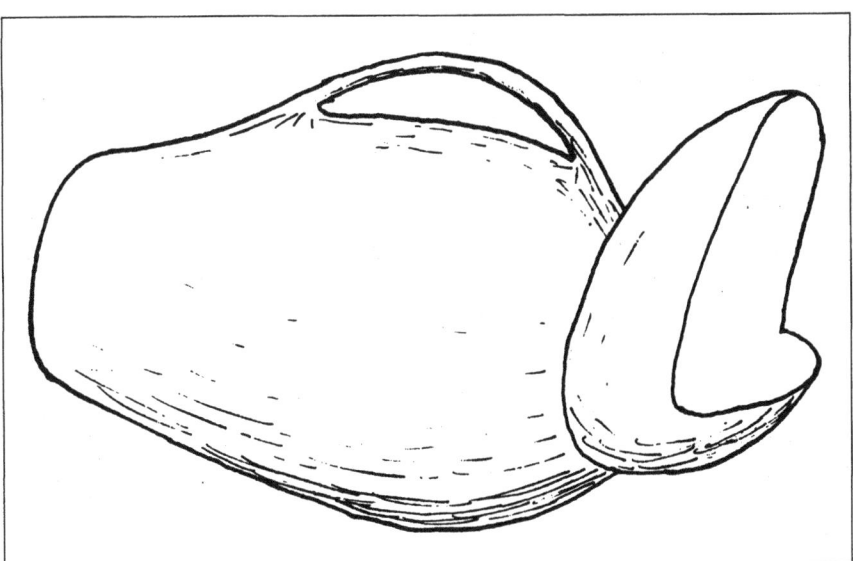

Figure 8–3 Urinal for Women

Important factors to consider when selecting a urinal are whether the design is appropriate for the position in which it will be used (e.g., sitting in a chair, standing, sitting in bed with the head elevated, in bed in the prone position); the shape of the neck to prevent leakage, especially when removing the urinal after voiding; and the shape of the neck of the urinal for comfortable and easy handling. As with the male urinal, the female urinal should be emptied regularly throughout the day, cleaned, and stored within easy reach of the older adult. A urinal should never be placed on the overbed table or any surface on which food is prepared for or consumed by the older adult. Not only is this unsanitary but it is demeaning to the individual.

Several portable devices are available for women to use in the standing or sitting positions (Help for Incontinent People, 1994). They are available in both reusable and disposable models. The woman either stands or sits, and voids into a funnel-like device, such as an artificial urethral extension, which can be attached to tubing and a collection bag or drained directly into a commode.

BEDPANS

The patent for the bedpan was issued in 1888, and its design has changed little over the years (Winslow, 1985). The bedpan was designed primarily for the convenience of the caregiver. Little research has been conducted regarding the benefits of the bedpan to the user. Two studies were conducted with normal subjects and individuals who had had a myocardial infarction. The researchers found that there was more oxygen and energy consumed and less patient satisfaction with the use of the bedpan than with out-of-bed toileting (Winslow, Lane, & Gaffney, 1984).

Bedpans come in two designs: the fracture bedpan and the regular bedpan (see Figures 8–4 and 8–5). The fracture pan was designed for individuals who are unable to lift their hips to position themselves on the bedpan. The handle allows the caregiver to remove the pan gently without turning or lifting the user. Proper placement of both types of bedpans under the body is imperative to avoid spills and leaks onto the bed. Extreme care should be taken to protect bony prominences and avoid shearing forces. For proper placement the individual should flex at the hips and lower the buttocks onto the pan, or be rolled from a lateral position onto the pan. The pan should never be forced under the buttocks, which can pull and possibly damage the skin. The head of the bed should be raised as high as the individual can tolerate while on the bedpan, to facilitate bladder emptying. No one should be left unattended on the bedpan for a prolonged period of time. A call light or bell should be left with the older adult so that help is readily available. Access to toilet tissue and a means to clean the hands are necessary as well. If the individual is unable to lift up onto the bedpan or roll onto it, then an overhead trapeze may

Supportive Devices for Urine Control 171

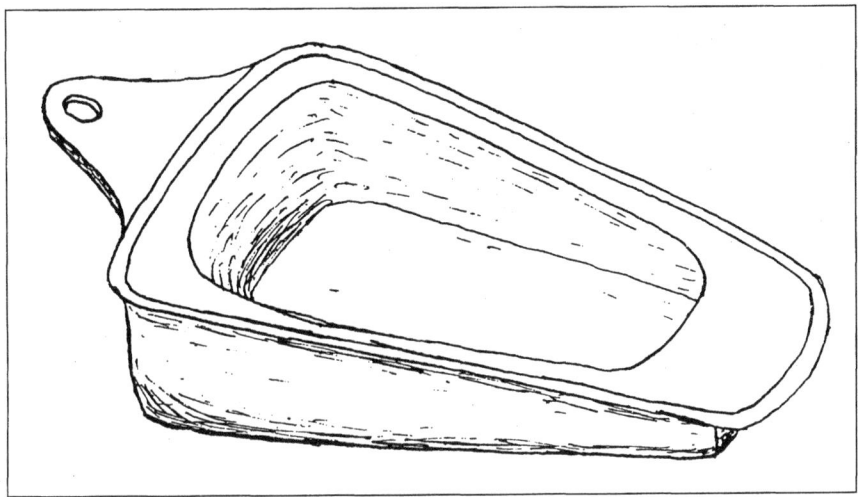

Figure 8–4 Fracture Bedpan

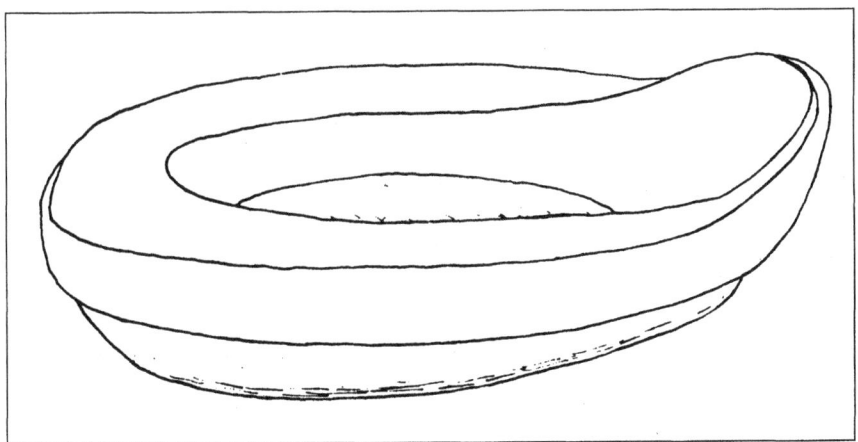

Figure 8–5 Regular Bedpan

be required. Besides patient safety and comfort, staff safety is another important consideration. Ergonomic interventions in the form of mechanical lifts can protect against back injury (Garg & Owen, 1992). Also, a reusable, waterproof, inflatable lift to raise the pelvis is available to help a caregiver slide a bedpan under the person without pulling at or damaging the skin (Kimbro, 1992).

EXTERNAL COLLECTION DEVICES FOR MEN

Disposable external collection devices for men have been available for several years. There are many styles on the market, and selection is dependent on individual need. Many of the condom catheters or sheaths are made of latex and should not be used on men with latex sensitivity. The skin of the penis should also be checked for irritation in men with no history of sensitivity. For men who are sensitive to latex, nonlatex condom catheters are available (Help for Incontinent People, 1994).

In order to have successful use of these devices, patient cooperation and education are necessary. Confused patients may pull off or displace the devices, and the tubing can become kinked in restless or ambulatory individuals. Because of this, these products may not be appropriate for confused and/or cognitively impaired older adults.

The collector should be changed at least once every day and proper skin care given. This includes inspection for irritation, cleansing, moisturizing, and protection (Faller & Jeter, 1992). When adhesive strips are used to apply the appliance, care should be taken not to constrict the penis. Impaired circulation from a too-tight condom or adhesive strip can lead to serious complications, including ulceration and necrosis.

The older adult should be encouraged, if possible, to learn how to apply the device and assess skin changes or problems. The collector may be connected to either a bedside drainage bag or a leg bag. The leg bag attaches with a garterlike strap to the lower leg and is worn under clothing, thus permitting ambulation. The bedside drainage bag, placed inside a cloth bag with a drawstring, should be positioned lower than the bladder at the side or at the foot of the bed. This permits easy inspection and emptying by health care providers while promoting the individual's privacy and self-image. The drainage bags must be emptied regularly to prevent dislodging the collector due to the weight of the urine, and must be cleaned or changed regularly to prevent odor and bacterial growth.

A penile clamp is another external device for men with slight urinary incontinence. The hazards of this device often outweigh the benefits. Damage to penile tissue, such as edema, ulceration, and stricture of the urethra, must be guarded against by using meticulous care. Men who are cognitively intact, are able to assess the skin for breakdown, and can articulate feelings of distress and the sensation of bladder fullness should be considered the only candidates for this device.

EXTERNAL COLLECTION DEVICES FOR WOMEN

Throughout history, attempts have been made to create an external collection device for women (Pieper, Cleland, Johnson, & O'Reilly, 1989). Pieper & Cleland (1993) described the complexities involved in the development of an external collection device for women. Currently, pouches that encircle the urethral opening and are secured by adhesive, pressure, or suction are available (Help for Incontinent People, 1994). Devices that incorporate a tube that is inserted into the urethra or vagina are available as well.

The noninvasive pouch has been used with older women and is applied by using an adhesive paste to the perineum. The opening of the pouch encircles the labia, urethral opening, and the vaginal introitus (Johnson, Muncie, O'Reilly, & Warren, 1990). It is difficult to apply this device on a woman unable to abduct her legs. For proper application, the mons pubis should be shaved. However, some women may object to being shaved and the discomfort caused by the regrowth of hair. This device, however, may be a viable alternative to an indwelling catheter or straight catheterization for specimen collection.

TIMING DEVICES

In the past, one timing device used in bladder training programs consisted of an alarm clock and a flashing light (Willington, 1976). At a preset time, the light flashed until it was switched off or until the batteries ran down. The purpose of this device was to remind the individual to go to the bathroom (Roe, 1977). The application of this device presumed that the older adult could interpret the message properly and ambulate to the bathroom with minimal assistance. Currently, watches are available that can be programmed to beep at a preset time. These can be used for the same purpose. Also, timing devices that emit sounds or light are available (Help for Incontinent People, 1994). Generally they are less intrusive and less stigmatizing than the older timing devices.

DAMPNESS DETECTORS

Another device to assist in bladder training is a dampness detector. When the individual voids and urine comes into contact with a sensor pad, the sensor pad signals a battery-operated clock to stop at the actual time of the incontinent incident (Ball & McFadden, 1975). This recorded information is important to caregivers keeping a voiding chart and developing a training program. Balmaseda, Fatehi, and Johnson (1984) described a micturition-alert device that was developed to detect voiding in people who are unable to detect the sensation of voiding but require having a postvoid residual calculated as part of their treatment plan. This device consists of a condom catheter, a sterile sensor located inside the condom, and a base unit that emits a piercing noise when urine comes into contact with the sensor. Enuresis detectors are readily available and are suitable for the home environment (Help for Incontinent People, 1994).

CLOTHING

Home health care medical supply catalogues offer an array of clothing for incontinent older adults. Velcro fasteners are used instead of snaps, buttons, and zippers for individuals with limited manual dexterity. Wraparound skirts with generous overlap are available for women to promote increased mobility and increase the ease in toileting (see Figure 8–6). Trousers with elasticized waists, to make pulling them down over the hips easier, are helpful to both women and men (Turnbull, 1985). Velcro zippers, drop seats, and extra-long zippers are helpful for the incontinent older man.

Clothing of quality design and construction that conceals the special adaptations it contains for urinary incontinence will bolster self-esteem, preserve dignity, and allow and encourage the individual to remain an active member of society. Attractive clothing also sends the message to the older adult that the caregiver respects and supports the right to be continent.

INDWELLING CATHETERS

Attempts to drain the bladder via a tube have been made for many centuries. There is evidence that reeds were used for this purpose in ancient China (Roe, 1991). In the 1930s Frederick Foley designed a rubber tube with a separate lumen used to inflate a balloon to hold the catheter in place in the bladder (Newman & Blackwood, 1991). The design of indwelling catheters has not changed radically since that time. Before the development of the closed system, in which the indwelling catheter and its connecting tubing are attached to a sealed drainage bag, catheters drained into open bottles or pails (Newman & Blackwood, 1991). With the open system, urinary tract infections were universal. In fact, even with the closed system and despite excellent hygiene, the majority of individuals who have

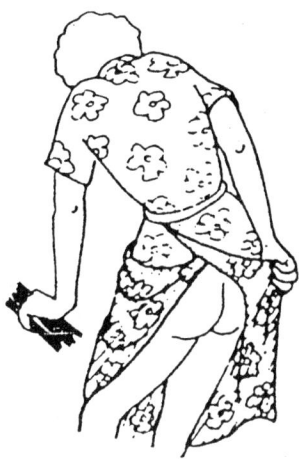

Figure 8–6 Clothing To Promote Continence. *Source:* Reprinted from Turnbull, P., Clothing for Independence, *Nursing Times*, Vol. 81, p. 55, with permission of Macmillan Magazines Ltd., © 1985.

---

an indwelling catheter are bacteriuric after 30 days. The best method of preventing an infection is by preventing the catheterization (Warren, 1990).

At one time, the indwelling catheter was considered the only equipment necessary for the treatment of chronic urinary incontinence. Unfortunately, some people are still of the opinion that it is the only sure solution. However, because of the prevalence of serious complications from long-term catheter usage, the indwelling catheter should be the last form of treatment considered for urinary incontinence. Change frequency for an indwelling catheter should be based on the individual's propensity to develop the complications listed in Exhibit 8–2.

Despite the complications associated with its use, the indwelling catheter does serve an important function. In situations where bladder decompression is needed, where there is an urgent need for accurate urinary output or protection of wounds or skin, and/or where there is serious renal dysfunction, an indwelling catheter may be an essential part of the treatment plan. Also, in cases of comatose or terminally ill individuals, when the benefits of comfort to the patient outweigh the risks of catheterization, the indwelling catheter may be the appropriate continence management option. However, the need for the indwelling catheter must be constantly re-evaluated and the catheter removed immediately when the need no longer exists.

Exhibit 8–2 Nursing Implications for Complications of Long-Term Catheter Placement

Complication	Nursing action
Irritation/pain/discomfort	Reduce catheter and balloon size. Anchor the catheter.
Inadvertent dislodgment	Assess for etiology of spasms (i.e., obstruction, catheter irritation, infection).
Obstruction	Implement a bowel program because fecal impaction/constipation causes blockage and leakage.
Catheter irritation	Use a bonded hydrogel catheter. Anchor the catheter. Use smaller catheter and balloon size. Limit number of catheter changes.
Infection	Use closed drainage system. Eliminate ambulatory drainage containers. Avoid catheter irrigators.
Encrustation	Check urine pH: pH > 5: acidify the urine by giving three 8-oz glasses of cranberry juice or 1 g of ascorbic acid per day. Increase fluid intake to eight 10-oz glasses per day. Increase frequency of catheter changes to prevent total blockage.

Source: Reprinted from Fiers, S., Indwelling Catheters and Devices: Avoiding the Problems, *Urologic Nursing*, Vol. 14, No. 3, p. 143, with permission of Mosby-Year Book, © 1994.

The use of the most appropriate catheter size (the smaller the better, usually 14F, 16F, or 18F) will help prevent distention of the urethra (Fiers, 1994). It is also recommended that a 5-ml balloon inflated to 10 ml be used to hold the catheter in the bladder without causing irritation and occlusion of the bladder neck (Fiers, 1994). An individual's sensitivity to latex should be noted, and a nonlatex catheter, usually a silicone catheter, should be used instead. Some catheters have a permanent bonded coating of hydrogel on both the inside and outside of the catheter, which helps to reduce the buildup of encrustations and reduce latex sensitivity (Newman & Blackwood, 1991).

Adequate hydration to keep the urine dilute, excellent hygiene that includes daily perineal care with a gentle cleanser, maintenance of the closed system with unobstructed flow, and meticulous equipment care are all essential elements for proper catheter maintenance (see Exhibit 8–3). Keeping the urine acidic by

Exhibit 8–3 Basic Care of Indwelling Catheters

Catheters should be inserted by trained personnel only, under aseptic conditions.

"Downhill" flow should always be maintained at all times (i.e., the collection bag should always be below the level of the patient's bladder).

Manipulation of catheters should be kept to a minimum.

Routine catheter irrigation and routine changing of the catheter are not helpful in preventing bacterial colonization.

Catheters may be irrigated if decreased flow is noted. If blockage is detected, the catheter should be changed.

When upper urinary tract infection or urinary sepsis is suspected, the catheter should be removed and a new catheter placed to obtain a specimen for culture. Bacteriuria is to be expected. Antibiotic prophylaxis or full treatment is not indicated for asymptomatic bacteriuria.

Source: Reprinted from Brechtelsbauer, D., Care with an Indwelling Urinary Catheter, *Postgraduate Medicine*, Vol. 92, No. 1, p. 128, with permission of McGraw-Hill, © 1992.

---

administering oral vitamin C has been suggested as one way to reduce the risk of a urinary tract infection (Roe, 1990). There is evidence that cranberry juice reduces bacterial adherence to the bladder wall (Rogers, 1991). Warren (1990) reported that irrigation of the catheter does not prevent infection. In fact, by breaking the closed system, introduction of pathogens could occur. The drainage bag should always be lower than the bladder, and it should never come into contact with the floor. Extra care must be taken when changing or repositioning the tubing so that back flow toward the bladder does not occur. Catheters do not need to be replaced routinely, unless the flow is reduced or the catheter is blocked (Brechtelsbauer, 1992).

Intermittent catheterization and self-catheterization are two measures that are possible alternatives to long-term catheter placement for some individuals, especially for those who have little or no bladder emptying due to trauma or neurogenic dysfunctions. Careful assessment of the individual's medical and functional status and ability to tolerate and perform catheterizations must be conducted. Sadowski and Duffy (1988) found that clean, intermittent catheterization is appropriate for some nursing home residents. However, *sterile* intermittent catheterization is recommended for elderly patients (Fantl, Newman, & Colling, et al., 1996).

Highly motivated older adults who are free of serious functional limitations and medical risk may be taught intermittent catheterization. Besides the physiological advantage of not having a chronic foreign object in the bladder, the psychological advantage is obvious. The individual is unencumbered by the constant presence of the tubing and a drainage bag. A sense of independence and concealment of a urologic disruption can add to the psychological well-being of the individual. Candidates for self-catheterization require cognitive skills to understand instructions and the rationale for the procedure, as well as the physical skills for inserting the catheter and cleaning it (see Exhibit 8–4).

CONCLUSION

Many products exist to improve the care of incontinent older adults. The successful application of devices depends on a thorough and individualized assessment. However, some general rules apply:

- Devices and equipment must be selected to best meet the individual's needs. This means that careful assessment of the underlying disruption, the severity of symptoms, and the expectations of the individual must first be performed.
- All devices and equipment must be kept in safe working order and cleaned and disinfected according to the manufacturer's instructions. Most companies supply information about proper use and maintenance of their products.
- The older adult and caregivers must receive instructions regarding the use and care of the devices and equipment. They should be questioned about their

---

Exhibit 8–4 General Guidelines for Clean, Intermittent Catheterization

> Have equipment ready—catheter, lubricant, mirror (some women need a mirror to locate the meatus).
>
> Wash hands with soap and water.
>
> While seated on the toilet (or standing, for men) wash the meatus, then lubricate the catheter (size 14F or 16F for women and 16F or 18F for men) with a water-soluble lubricant.
>
> Insert the catheter through the urethral meatus into the bladder (5 to 7.5 cm for women, 15 to 25 cm for men).
>
> Remove the catheter after emptying bladder, and clean it with soap and water. Rinse thoroughly.
>
> Remove excess water from the catheter and store the catheter in plastic bag or container.
>
> *Note:* Clean, intermittent catheterization is performed by the older adult approximately every 3 to 6 hours per day. Fluid intake of 2,400 ml per day is recommended.

understanding of the product's use, its limitations, and realistic performance expected of the equipment.
- Devices and equipment must never replace the human element of care. Caregivers must be aware of the psychological effects of incontinence products on the user and provide empathetic concern. Sharp assessment and observation skills on the part of caregivers are still necessary to prevent complications, such as skin breakdown and infection, and to maintain the quality of care and life of the individual.

New products are constantly introduced in the market. The caregiver must keep abreast of the latest literature regarding these products and discuss the advantages and disadvantages of these products with other caregivers and the incontinent older adult.

Careful assessment of urinary incontinence must be performed before any device or equipment to enhance urine control is selected and employed. The older adult's needs and concerns must be addressed during the decision-making process. The device or equipment should promote the older adult's self-esteem and physical comfort. The benefits must outweigh the risks. No product should be used as a substitute for human contact with the caregivers.

REFERENCES

Ball, J., & McFadden, M. (1975). A dampness detector for use with incontinent patients. *British Medical Journal, 3*, 466–467.

Balmaseda, M., Fatehi, M., & Johnson, E. (1984). Micturition alert device. *Archives of Physical Medical Rehabilitation, 65*, 554–555.

Bierwirth, W. (1992). Which pad is for you? *Urologic Nursing, 12*(2), 75–77.

Brechtelsbauer, D. (1992). Care with an indwelling urinary catheter. *Postgraduate Medicine, 92*, 127–132.

Brink, C., & Wells, T. (1986). Environmental support for geriatric incontinence. *Clinics in Geriatric Medicine, 2*, 829–840.

Clancy, B. (1989). Bed protectors: No easy choices. *Nursing Times, 85*(33), 71–72.

Clancy, B., & Malone-Lee, J. (1991). Reducing the leakage of body-worn incontinence pads. *Journal of Advanced Nursing, 16*, 187–193.

Cottenden, A. (1988). Incontinence pads and appliances. *International Disabilities Studies, 10*, 44–47.

Faller, N., & Jeter, K. (1992). The ABCs of product selection. *Urologic Nursing, 12*(2), 52–54.

Fantl, J.A., Newman, D.K., & Colling, J. et al. (1996). *Urinary incontinence in adults: Acute and chronic management. Clinical practice guideline no. 2, 1996 update.* (AHCPR Pub. No. 96-0692). Rockville, MD: Agency for Health Care Policy and Research, Public Health Service, U.S. Department of Health and Human Services.

Fiers, S. (1994). Indwelling catheters and devices: Avoiding the problems. *Urologic Nursing, 14*(3), 141–144.

Garg, A., & Owen, B. (1992). Reducing back stress to nursing personnel: An ergonomic intervention in a nursing home. *Ergonomics, 35,* 1353–1375.

Help for Incontinent People. (1994). *Resource guide* (6th ed.). Union, SC: Author.

Johnson, D., Muncie, H., O'Reilly, J., & Warren, J. (1990). An external urine collection device for incontinent women. *Journal of the American Geriatrics Society, 38,* 1016–1022.

Kimbro, C. (1992). A caregiver technology advance. *International Journal of Technology and Aging, 5,* 179–185.

Newman, D., & Blackwood, N. (1991). Applications and perspectives on the use of indwelling catheters. Presented at The National Multi-Specialty Nursing Conference, Kissimmee, Florida, November 20, 1991.

Pieper, B., & Cleland, V. (1993). An external urine-collection device for women: A clinical trial. *Journal of ET Nursing, 20,* 51–55.

Pieper, B., Cleland, V., Johnson, D., & O'Reilly, J. (1989). Inventing urine incontinence devices for women. *Image, 21,* 205–209.

Pottle, B. (1986). When the sheets were changed. *Nursing Times, 82,* 64, 66.

Roe, B. (1977). Incontinence timing devices. *Age and Ageing, 6,* 238–239.

Roe, B. (1990). Catheter prescribing and the use of antimicrobials. *Nursing Times, 86*(14), 65–68.

Roe, B. (1991). Looking at the evidence. *Nursing Times, 87*(37), 72, 74.

Rogers, J. (1991). Pass the cranberry juice. *Nursing Times, 87*(48), 36–37.

Sadowski, A., & Duffy, L. (1988). A survey of clean intermittent catheterization in long term care. *Urologic Nursing, 8,* 15–17.

Turnbull, P. (1985). Clothing for independence. *Nursing Times, 81,* 55–57, 63.

Warren, J. (1990). Urine-collection devices for use in adults with urinary incontinence. *Journal of the American Geriatrics Society, 38,* 364–367.

Willington, F. L. (1969). Problems in urinary incontinence in the aged. *Gerontologia Clinicia, 11,* 330–356.

Willington, F. L. (1976). *Incontinence in the elderly.* New York: Academic Press.

Winslow, E. (1985). Overcautious use of the bedpan. *American Journal of Nursing, 85,* 643–644.

Winslow, E., Lane, L., & Gaffney, A. (1984). Oxygen uptake and cardiovascular response in patients and normal adults during in-bed and out-of-bed toileting. *Journal of Cardiac Rehabilitation, 4,* 348–354.

APPENDIX

A

Glossary

Activities of Daily Living (ADLs)—Activities necessary to meet essential human needs, such as bathing, grooming, toileting, and social interactions.

Afferent nerve pathways—Sensory nerve pathways carrying nerve impulses toward the spinal cord and brain.

Alpha-adrenergic agonists—Medications that stimulate physiological activity of alpha-adrenergic receptors. These medications stimulate urethral resistance and are used in the treatment of stress incontinence.

Alpha-adrenergic blockers—Medications that block the activity of alpha-adrenergic receptors. Because these medications can decrease urethral resistance, stress incontinence may occur.

Alzheimer's disease—Progressive neuropsychiatric disease causing irreversible cognitive dysfunction and eventual physical impairment.

Anticholinergic—A medication or agent that blocks or impedes the actions of parasympathetic nerves; emptying of the bladder is primarily a parasympathetic activity. Therefore, anticholinergics facilitate storage by increasing bladder capacity and decreasing bladder contractions.

Atonic bladder—Also referred to as a lower motor neuron bladder. Often caused by peripheral neuropathies, such as diabetes mellitus. The bladder is flaccid and overdistended with urine. Overflow incontinence may occur.

Bacteriuria—Bacteria present in the urine. Bacteriuria is considered significant when there are $\geq 10^5$ colonies of pathogens in 1 ml of urine and the person complains of burning, frequency, flank pain, or other symptoms of infection. Signs of significant bacteriuria in older adults include change in temperature, changes in ability to perform ADLs or in functional status, and delirium.

Bedside commode—A portable toilet used by individuals who have difficulty ambulating to standard toilet facilities.

Benign prostatic hyperplasia (BPH)—Noncancerous enlargement of the prostate gland. More than 50% of men over the age of 60 years have BPH. BPH may have irritative or obstructive urinary symptoms.

Biofeedback—A technique to provide auditory or visual information to an individual about a specific physiological process. Biofeedback is used in the behavioral treatment of incontinence.

Bladder—A collapsible muscular organ of the lower urinary tract. The bladder acts as a reservoir for urine.

Bladder training—Also known as bladder retraining or re-education. The principle of bladder training is to increase the time span between voidings by encouraging the individual to suppress the urge to void for a period of time. The goal of bladder training is to achieve as normal a pattern of micturition as possible. It is used in the treatment of urge incontinence.

Calculi—Also called stones. Calculi may form in the bladder, ureters, and kidneys.

Catheter—A tube inserted into the body to inject or draw off fluids. An indwelling catheter is a tube inserted through the urethra to the bladder to drain off urine continuously.

Cerebral cortex—The site of conscious control of micturition. The cortical center of control situated in the frontal lobes is located in the cerebral cortex.

Cerebrovascular accident (CVA)—Most often caused by a thrombosis or embolus in a cerebral artery, causing damage to brain tissue.

Continence—The ability to control the act of urination.

Cortical center of control—*See* Cerebral cortex.

Cystitis—Inflammation of the bladder. Symptoms include painful and frequent urination.

Cystocele—Prolapse of the bladder through the anterior vaginal wall. Prolapses are staged, using objective criteria, by the severity of the maximum protrusion of the prolapse during examination.

Cystometrogram (CMG)—An invasive test used to assess bladder function. Sterile water or sterile saline is introduced into the bladder. The sensation of the need to void, bladder pressure, and bladder contractions are measured in relation to volume.

Cystourethrocele—A prolapse of the bladder and the urethra.

Defecation—The act of emptying the bowels.

Delirium—An acute confusional state that develops rapidly but may take weeks to resolve. A reduced ability to shift or maintain attention to stimuli outside the individual and disorganized thinking are cardinal signs.

Dementia—A term used for an impairment in short- and long-term memory. There are also impairments in abstract thinking, judgment, and impulse control.

Dependent continence—The individual is kept continent solely through the efforts of the nursing staff.

Detrusor—Smooth muscle of the bladder. Stretches to accommodate and store urine and contracts uniformly to empty.

Detrusor hyperactivity with impaired contractility (DHIC)—Frequent bladder contractions occur but are ineffective in completely emptying the bladder. The individual usually has a high postvoid residual.

Detrusor sphincter dyssynergia (DSD)—Lack of coordination between detrusor contraction and sphincter relaxation and contraction.

Distal urethral sphincter mechanism—A term used to describe the portion of the urethra farthest from the bladder; located in the perineum of a woman and in the glans of a man's penis.

Diuretic—An agent that increases urination.

Dysuria—Difficulty in urination.

Efferent nerve pathways—These nerves carry impulses away from the brain, causing muscles to contract or to inhibit an organ. Also referred to as motor nerves.

Electrical stimulation—Treatment of urinary incontinence by providing electrical stimulation of the pelvic viscera and nerve.

Enterocele—Prolapses of small intestine into the pouch of Douglas, an area between the rectum and the vagina.

Enuresis—Urinary incontinence. Also used when describing nighttime incontinence (e.g., nighttime enuresis).

Established incontinence—Pattern of incontinence that is chronic in nature. There are several types of established incontinence: urge, stress, overflow, and functional.

Estrogen—Female sex hormone. Estrogen is used in postmenopausal women in a topical, oral, or patch form to alleviate urogenital atrophy that occurs from aging and to increase vascularization of tissue.

Fecal impaction—Large amount of hardened stool in the rectum that an individual is unable to pass. A fecal impaction may present as small amounts of watery and incontinent stool. Overflow incontinence can be caused by a fecal impaction.

Frequency—A symptom of urinary dysfunction, characterized by small-volume voidings in short time intervals.

Functional incontinence—Occurs in individuals who can control micturition, but factors outside the urinary tract cause incontinence. These factors include lack of access to toilets, immobility, and cognitive and psychological impairments.

Habit training—Assistance to the toilet or use of bedpan or urinal offered based on the individual's voiding pattern.

Hematuria—Blood in the urine.

Hormone replacement therapy—Provision of estrogen to postmenopausal women to treat symptoms of menopause and urinary incontinence, to protect the cardiovascular system, and to prevent osteoporosis. Estrogen may be given alone or in conjunction with progesterone.

Hyper-reflexia—A term used to describe the abnormal contraction of the detrusor in the presence of a neurological cause, such as a cerebrovascular accident.

Hypogastric plexus—An area in the spinal cord, between T-11 and L-2, that receives afferent information about bladder fullness. It is also the site of efferent sympathetic nerve activity, facilitating bladder storage.

Incontinence—*See* Urinary incontinence.

Increased afferent loop stimulation—A term used to describe the abnormally rapid transmission of and reception of afferent impulses overwhelming the cortical center's ability to inhibit detrusor contractions. Causes include irritants to the bladder wall, such as a urinary tract infection or an enlarged prostate.

Independent continence—The individual is able to maintain continence without assistance.

Intermittent catheterization (IC)—An alternative to long-term catheterization for individuals with reflex incontinence. IC promotes the independence of older adults and reduces the chances of acquiring a urinary tract infection.

Intraurethral pressure—Pressure within the urethra. An important component in maintaining continence.

Intravesical pressure—Pressure within the bladder.

Kegel exercises—Exercises named after Dr. Kegel, who first prescribed a specific set of pelvic floor exercises to postpartum women in the 1940s. These exercises are also called pelvic muscle exercises.

Kidneys—Bean-shaped organs of the renal system. Urine forms in the kidneys and travels through the ureters to the bladder.

Levator ani—The muscles that provide the structural support of the pelvic floor. These muscles surround the urethra and vagina. The pubococcygeus is the most important of the three muscles that comprise the levator ani.

Lithotomy position—The individual is placed on the back with thighs abducted and legs flexed.

Lower center of control—Sacral reflex center located in the sacral area of the spinal cord. Responsible for transmitting signals to the detrusor to expand or contract and to the cortical center of control of the need to void.

Lower neuron lesions—Lesions in the sacral reflex center or lower causing disruptions in the emptying of the bladder, such as overflow incontinence.

Manometry—A technique to measure the pressure or tension within the bladder.

Micturition—The act of urination.

Minimum data set (MDS)—A federally mandated screening and assessment form for Medicare- and Medicaid-certified long-term care facilities in the United States. This form is completed within 14 days of admission to the facility, quarterly, and when there is a significant change in the resident's status. An annual update is also required. The information collected in the MDS is used in planning the care of the individual.

Multi-infarct dementia—Deterioration of mental faculties from small infarcted areas in the brain. Affected individuals usually have a history of hypertension, previous CVAs, or vascular disease.

Multiple sclerosis—A demyelinating neurological disease leading to decline in function in the organs affected by the lesions in the nerve pathways.

Myopathic—Disease of a muscle.

Nocturia—Urination during the night.

Nulliparous—Never having given birth to a live baby.

Overflow incontinence—Involuntary loss of urine associated with an overdistended bladder.

Palpation—A technique of physical examination. The palmar surface of the fingers is used to delineate organs and masses and to detect tenderness.

Parasympathetic activity—Emptying of the bladder is mainly a parasympathetic activity. The parasympathetic nervous system is a division of the autonomic nervous system. The sacral outflow nerves are part of the parasympathetic (cholinergic) nervous system.

Parkinson's disease—A progressive neurological disease characterized by symptoms of muscle rigidity, tremor, and impaired mobility.

Partial continence—The individual is dry the majority of the time through the efforts of the nursing staff or caregiver to help the individual retain urine within the body until it is time to empty the bladder.

Penis—Contains the male urethra and urinary meatus. Part of the urinary and reproductive systems of the male.

Perineum—The area between the vulva and anus in the female and the area between the scrotum and anus in men.

Peripheral neuropathy—Noninflammatory lesion anywhere in the peripheral nervous system. It can be caused by a thiamine deficiency as in alcoholic neuropathy or by diabetes mellitus.

Polyuria—Excretion of a large volume of urine during a certain interval of time. It can be a result of uncontrolled diabetes mellitus or the administration of a diuretic.

Pontine mesencephalic gray matter—Located in the brain stem and is responsible for the coordination of the relaxation of the sphincters and relaxation of the bladder.

Postvoid residual (PVR)—Urine remaining in the bladder after urination. *See* Residual urine.

Precipitancy—A short period of time between the knowledge of the need to void and the release of urine.

Pressure ulcers—A skin lesion caused by unrelieved pressure resulting in damage to the underlying tissues. Pressure ulcers are staged by degree of damage. Other terms that have been used are bedsores, decubitus, and pressure sores.

Prevalence—The number of causes of a disease or condition in a group of people at a certain point in time.

Prolapse—A dropping or protrusion of an organ.

Prompted voiding—A behavioral modification technique using verbal and physical cues to assist the individual to use the toilet.

Prostate gland—A gland in a man's urogenital tract surrounding the bladder neck and proximal portion of the urethra.

Prostatic hyperplasia (formerly prostatic hypertrophy)—Enlargement of the prostate gland commonly occurring in men after age 50. *See* Benign prostatic hyperplasia.

Proteinuria—The presence of excess serum protein in the urine. It may indicate renal disease.

Proximal urethra—The portion of the urethra closest to the bladder.

Psychotropics—Medications that affect the mental status. These include antidepressants and antipsychotics.

Pubococcygeus—Portion of the levator ani targeted for strengthening when pelvic muscle exercises are performed.

Rectocele—An outpouching of the rectal wall. The outpouching is evident on straining and defecation. The person may experience a sensation of incomplete rectal emptying.

Reflex incontinence—A term sometimes used to describe the incontinence due to the severance of the conscious control of micturition, resulting in inefficient emptying of the bladder.

Resident Assessment Profile (RAP)—Part of the minimum data set that assists the nurse to assess the cause of various disruptions or conditions. The RAP provides a systematic method of assessment and is used in the development of the care plan for the individual.

Residual urine—The amount of urine left in the bladder after an individual voids. Individuals with residual urine over 200 ml may have ineffective bladder emptying and may be at risk for developing urinary tract infections due to the stasis of urine.

Sacral reflex center—Also known as the lower center of control. The sacral reflex center is located S-2 to S-4 in the spinal cord.

Scheduled toileting—Assistance to toilet or use of bedpan or urinal offered on a fixed schedule, for example, every 2 to 4 hours.

Social continence—Continence is achieved only through containment measures, such as absorbent products.

Sphincter—Muscle designed to reduce or constrict the size of an opening.

Sphincter incompetence—A term used to describe a neurological or non-neurological cause of the sphincter to function ineffectively, thus affecting bladder storage.

Stress incontinence—Disruption caused by a sudden increase in intra-abdominal pressure with a corresponding increase in the intravesical pressure. Poor pelvic muscle tone and urethral sphincter weakness are associated with stress incontinence.

Sympathetic nervous system—Part of the autonomic nervous system. Its fibers originate in the thoracic and lumbar region of the spinal cord. Storage of urine is primarily a sympathetic activity.

Symphysis pubis—Also referred to as the pubic bone. The symphysis pubis is located posterior to the mon pubis.

Transient incontinence—Incontinence that occurs in a normally continent individual, occurring from a potentially reversible cause.

Trigone—Triangle-shaped muscle that extends up from the urethra up the posterior bladder wall to the ureteral openings.

Uninhibited bladder contractions—Also referred to as uninhibited detrusor. Contractions of the detrusor occur in the absence of conscious control.

Unstable detrusor—Uninhibited bladder contractions in the absence of a neurological cause.

Upper neuron lesions—Suprasacral lesions that disrupt the storage of urine.

Urge incontinence—Involuntary control of urine associated with a strong urge to void.

Ureters—Tubes that carry urine from the kidneys to the bladder.

Urethra—A tube leading from the base of the bladder to the exterior. It is approximately 1 to 1½ inches long in a woman and approximately 8 inches long in a man.

Urethral pressure profile—An assessment tool to measure the pressure along the length of the urethra.

Urethritis—Inflammation of the urethra.

Urethrocele—Prolapse of the urethra in women.

Urethrovesical—Junction of the urethra and bladder.

Urethrovesical angle—An angle formed by the urethra and the base of the bladder neck. Normally about 90 to 100 degrees in women. The loss of this angle is associated with stress incontinence.

Urgency—Heightened sensation of the need to void. Often urgency is a symptom of a urinary tract infection.

Urinal—A portable receptacle for urine usually made of plastic or metal. Versions for men and women are available.

Urinary incontinence—The involuntary loss of urine that is sufficient enough to be a problem.

Urinary meatus—Exterior opening of the urethra. The urinary meatus is located in the glans of the penis in men and in the perineum anterior to the vaginal opening in women.

Urinary retention—The condition in which an individual is unable to pass urine. Urinary retention can be secondary to medications, disruptions in innervation of the bladder, and/or outlet obstruction.

Urinary tract infection (UTI)—Infection in the urinary tract caused by an organism. Symptoms include burning, frequency, and dysuria.

Urination—The act of passing urine.

Uroflowmeter—A noninvasive test to measure the adequacy of urine flow. Disruptions in bladder emptying can be detected.

Vagina—Also known as the birth canal. The vagina is a collapsible tube of smooth muscle with its opening located between the urethral orifice and anal sphincter of women.

Vaginitis—Inflammation of the vagina characterized by itching and a yellowish or pinkish discharge.

Vesica—Term for a bladder or sac containing fluid.

Voiding—Passing urine, micturating, urinating.

APPENDIX

B

Additional Sources of Information

The information provided in this appendix is not meant to be all-inclusive but representative of further sources of information.

Nursing and Gerontological Journals

American Journal of Nursing
Geriatric Nursing
Gerontologist
Journal of the American Geriatrics Society
Journal of Gerontological Nursing
Journal of Wound, Ostomy, and Continence Nursing
Orthopaedic Nursing
Rehabilitation Nursing Research
Urologic Nursing

Professional Organizations

American Geriatrics Society
770 Lexington Avenue, Suite 300
New York, NY 10021

American Urogynecologic Society
P.O. Box 809277
Chicago, IL 60680-9277

Gerontological Society of America
1275 K Street, NW, Suite 350
Washington, DC 20005-4006

Society of Urologic Nurses and Associates
SUNA National Office
East Holly Avenue, Box 56
Pittman, NJ 08071-0056

Wound, Ostomy, and Continence Nursing
WOCN National Office
2755 Bristol Street, Suite 110
Costa Mesa, CA 92626

Organizations with Information About Urinary Incontinence

Bladder Health Council
Dept. P
300 W. Pratt Street
Baltimore, MD 21201-2463

Help for Incontinent People (HIP)
P.O. Box 8306
Spartansburg, SC 29305-8306
(800) BLADDER

The Simon Foundation
Box 815
Wilmette, IL 60091
(800) 23 SIMON

The National Institutes of Health
9000 Rockville Pike
Bethesda, MD 20892
Information Office
(301) 496-4000

Agency for Health Care Policy and Research
2101 East Jefferson Street
Suite 501
Rockville, MD 20852
(800) 358-9295
Instant FAX (301) 594-2800

Alliance for Aging Research
2021 K Street NW
Washington, DC 20006
(800) 497-0360

Index

A

Activities of daily living (ADLs), 54, 67, 181
Acute care setting
    assessment of incontinence in, 62–76
    prevalence of incontinence in, 28
    treatment of incontinence in, 107
Administrative issues, 129, 155
Agency for Health Care Policy and Research (AHCPR), 14, 86, 192
Age-related physiological changes, 10–12, 125–126
Alcohol, 42–43
Alcoholic neuropathy, 39
Alliance for Aging Research, 192
Alpha-adrenergic agonists, 41, 97, 99, 131, 181
Alpha-adrenergic blockers, 41, 138, 181
Alpha-adrenergic receptors, 96, 100
Alzheimer's disease, 146, 147, 148, 181
American Geriatrics Society, 190
American Urogynecologic Society, 190
Anger, 114
Anticholinergic drugs, 40, 41, 92, 96–98, 97, 181
Antidepressants, 42, 92, 97, 99
Antihistamines, 41, 42
Antiparkinsonian drugs, 41, 42
Antispasmodics, 41
Anxiety, 86
Assessment of incontinence, 47–76, 80–85
    in acute care setting, 62–76
        bowel and urogenital functioning, 65
        cognitive assessment, 63, 64
        medications, 65
        physical examination, 65–69, 71
        urinalysis, 69–70, 72–73
        urodynamic evaluation, 70–76
        voiding record, 62–63
    continence assessment form, 49–51
    in long-term care setting, 51–56
        algorithm for, 58
        delirium, 53
        depression, 55
        further assessment, 55–56, 57
        medical conditions, 53–55
        medications, 53
        Minimum Data Set, 51, 52
        mobility, 53
        Resident Assessment Profile, 51
        toilet facilities, 55
    in noninstitutionalized older adults, 56–62
        caregiver and living environment evaluation, 61–62
        history taking, 56, 59–60
        older adults' responses to assessment, 56–61
    role of nurses in, 47–51
Attitudes about continence, 154–156

B

Bacteriuria, 54–55, 69–70, 181
Bathing, 111–112
Bed protectors, 166

Bedpans, 170–172
Bedside commode, 168, 182
Behavioral Supervision Model, 94, 106
Behavioral treatments, 86–95
  behavioral modification, 91
  bladder training, 91–92
  electrical stimulation, 94–95
  habit training, 92–93
  in long-term care setting, 105–106
  pelvic floor training, 87–90
  prompted voiding, 93–94
  scheduled toileting, 92
  supportive devices and, 162
Benign prostatic hyperplasia (BPH), 182. *See also* Prostatic hyperplasia
Beta-adrenergic receptors, 96
Biofeedback, 88, 90, 182
Bladder, 1–3, 182
  anatomy of, 2, 4
  atonic, 20, 39, 181
  central neurogenic, 17
  changes with aging, 11
  innervation of, 2
  measuring filling of, 74–76
  spastic, 17
  stretch receptors of, 35, 39
  uninhibited contractions of, 9, 74, 188
  uninhibited neurogenic, 17
  unstable, 17
Bladder Health Council, 191
Bladder training, 91–92, 162, 182
Bowel function, 65, 149
Brain injury, 37
Briefs, absorbent, 163–166
  disposable, 163–164
  reusable, 164–166
Bromocriptine mesylate, 42
Brompheniramine maleate, 42
Bulbocavernosus reflex, 69

C

Calcium channel blockers, 41, 96
Calculi, 182
Care plans, 124
  for man with benign prostatic hyperplasia, 139–141
  for older adult with functional incontinence secondary to dementia, 150–151
  for older man with transient incontinence secondary to delirium, 144–146
  for postmenopausal woman with stress urinary incontinence, 134–136
Caregivers
  assessment of, 61–62
  psychological impact of incontinence to, 118–119
Catheter, 182
Catheterization
  intermittent, 96, 100–101, 177–178, 184
  suprapubic, 101
Causes of incontinence, 25, 30–44, 80–85
  environmental factors, 40–43
    alcohol, 42–43
    clothing, 43
    medications, 40–42
    toilet facilities, 43
  neurological factors, 35–39
    increased afferent loop stimulation, 39
    sacral spinal lesions, 39
    suprasacral spinal lesions, 37–39
  transient incontinence, 30
  urogenital factors, 31–35
    detrusor hyperactivity with impaired contractility, 34–35
    hormonal influences in women, 34
    pelvic floor weakness in women, 33–34
    pelvic prolapse in women, 32–33
    prostatic enlargement, 31–32
    urinary tract infection, 35
Cerebral cortex, 8, 182
  lesions of, 37–38
Cerebrovascular accident (CVA), 37, 182
Cholinergic receptors, 96
Clothing, 43, 101, 174, 175
Cognitive assessment, 63, 64, 86
Cognitive care, 131, 133, 137, 142, 147–148
Cognitive impairment. *See* Dementia
Communication, 86–87
  nonverbal, 146–147
Confusion, 40
Congestive heart failure (CHF), 53–54
Continence, 1, 7, 182
  dependent, 105–106, 155, 183
  independent, 105, 155, 184
  partial, 106–107, 155, 186
  philosophy of, 123–124, 127
  social, 105, 107, 155, 188
Continence program, 152–157
  antecedents to, 152, 153–154
  attitudes and beliefs for, 154–156
  barriers to, 157

evaluation of, 156
organizational issues in, 156
planning of, 157
Coping mechanisms, 86
Coping with Urinary Incontinence scale, 61
Cortical center of control, 8
Credé maneuver, 100, 104, 137
Cystitis, 182
Cystocele, 33, 69, 182
Cystometrogram (CMG), 74–76, 182
Cystourethrocele, 33, 183

D

Dampness protectors, 173–174
Defecation, 183
Delirium, 53, 103, 138, 183
   assessment for, 138, 141, 149, 152
   causes of, 138
   nursing care for older man with transient incontinence secondary to, 138, 142–143
   prevention of, 138
Dementia, 25, 38, 138, 146, 183
   Alzheimer's disease, 146, 147, 148, 181
   multi-infarct, 146, 147, 185
   nursing care of older adult with functional incontinence secondary to, 146–149
   vascular, 146
Depression, 55, 67, 99, 114, 148
Detrusor muscle, 2, 9, 183
   hyperactivity with impaired contractility (DHIC), 34–35, 98, 183
   hyper-reflexia of, 17, 37, 39
   unstable, 17, 188
Diabetes mellitus, 39, 53–54
DIAPPERS acronym, 30, 102
Dicyclomine hydrochloride, 99
Disopyramide, 41
Diuretics, 40, 41, 54, 183
Douching, 132
Doxepin hydrochloride, 42, 99
DRIP acronym, 30, 102
Dysuria, 65, 183

E

Education, 125–127, 158
Electrical stimulation, 94–95, 183
Electromyography, 88
Embarrassment, 60, 70, 114, 127
Empathy, 132

Enterocele, 33, 183
Enuresis, 183
Environmental assessment, 61–62, 67
Environmental influences, 40–43, 101, 106, 128
Environmental modifications, 101, 106, 128, 166–167
Ephedrine, 99
Escherichia coli infection, 102
Estrogen, 10, 34, 97, 99–100, 131, 184
External collection devices, 172–173

F

Falling, fear of, 166
FANCAPES acronym, 138, 141
Fecal impaction, 35, 39, 103, 149, 184
Finasteride, 138
Fluid intake, 105, 133
Folstein "Mini-Mental State" Examination, 64
Frequency, 53, 65, 184
Frustration, 86
Functional assessment screening, 66–68

G

Gerontological Society of America, 191
Glaucoma, 98
Glycosuria, 69
Graves speculum, 55
Grief, 114
Guideline for Urinary Incontinence in Adults, 14

H

Habit training, 92–93, 162, 184
Hearing screening, 66
Help for Incontinent People (HIP), 191
Hematuria, 56, 69, 184
History taking, 56, 59–60
Home care setting
   assessment of incontinence in, 56–62
   prevalence of incontinence in, 28
   treatment of incontinence in, 107
Hopelessness, 86, 117
Hormone replacement therapy, 131, 184
Hygiene habits, 70, 86, 117
   historical perspective on, 111–114
Hyper-reflexia, 17, 37, 39, 184
Hypogastric plexus, 3, 8, 184

I

Imipramine hydrochloride, 99
Incontinence Impact Questionnaire, 117
Incontinence Stress Questionnaire-Patient (ISQ-P), 117–118
Increased afferent loop stimulation, 39, 184
Indwelling catheters, 101, 107, 174–177
Intermittent catheterization, 96, 100–101, 177–178, 184

K

Kegel exercises, 86, 87–90, 131, 185
Kidneys, 1, 185
  changes with aging, 10–11
Kylie sheet, 166

L

Levator ani muscle, 4–5, 87, 185
Lithotomy position, 56, 185
Long-term care setting
  assessment of incontinence in, 51–56
  nursing care in, 123–158
  prevalence of incontinence in, 25, 27, 104
  setting up continence program in, 152–157
  staff training in, 106
  treatment of incontinence in, 104–107
Lower center of control, 185
Lower neuron lesions, 185

M

Manometry, 88, 185
Marsupial pant, 164, 165
Medications affecting continence, 40–42, 53, 65, 104
Medications to treat incontinence, 96–100
  side effects of, 96, 97
  sites of action of, 96, 98
Mental status examination, 63, 64, 67
Micturition, 1–12
  age effects on, 10–12
  cortical center of control for, 8
  cycle of, 8–10
  definition of, 185
  role of bladder and urethra in, 1–6
  role of kidneys and ureters in, 1
  role of spinal cord in, 6–8
  structural components of, 36
  voluntary control of, 35
Minimum Data Set (MDS), 51, 52, 102, 104, 185
Mitral valve prolapse, 76
Mobility assessment, 53
Motivation, 86
Mourning, 114
Multiple sclerosis, 69, 185
Muscle relaxants, 97, 99
Muscular changes with aging, 11–12
Myopathy, 185

N

Narcotics, 41
National Institutes of Health, 191
Nerve pathways
  afferent, 8, 39, 181
  efferent, 8, 183
  increased afferent loop stimulation, 39, 184
Neurological changes with aging, 11
Neurological factors affecting continence, 35–39
Nocturia, 185
Nulliparous, 186
Nursing assistants, 155
Nursing care, 123–158
  assessment of incontinence, 47–51
  goals of, 124, 125
  of man with benign prostatic hyperplasia, 133–138
    cognitive care, 133, 137
    physical care, 137–138
    psychological care, 137
    sample care plan, 139–141
  of older adult with functional incontinence secondary to dementia, 146–149
    cognitive care, 147–148
    physical care, 149
    psychological care, 148
    sample care plan, 150–151
  of older man with transient incontinence secondary to delirium, 138, 142–143
    cognitive care, 142
    physical care, 143
    psychological care, 142–143
    sample care plan, 144–146

philosophy of continence, 123–124, 127, 153
of postmenopausal woman with stress urinary incontinence, 131–136
  cognitive care, 131
  physical care, 132–133
  psychological care, 131–132
  sample care plan, 134–136
psychological impact of incontinence, 119–120
setting up a continence program, 152–157
  antecedents to, 152, 153–154
  attitudes and beliefs, 154–156
  barriers, 157
  evaluation, 156
  organizational issues, 156
  planning, 157
standards of, 124, 156
Nursing journals, 190
Nursing roles, 125–130
Nutritional assessment, 66

O

Obstetrical history, 65
Orientation, 40, 142
Oxybutynin chloride, 99

P

Pad test, 73
Pads, absorbent, 163–166
Palpation, 69, 186
Parasympathetic activity, 8, 96, 186
Parkinson's disease, 41, 42, 69, 186
Pathophysiology of incontinence, 29
Patterned urge-response toileting (PURT), 92–93
Pederson speculum, 55
Pelvic floor muscles, 4, 8
  training of, 87–90, 126, 131
  weakness in women, 33–34
Pelvic prolapse in women, 32–33, 55, 56, 186
Penile clamp, 172–173
Penis, 69, 186
Perineal care, 105, 128, 143
Perineometer, 87
Perineum, 186
Peripheral neuropathy, 39, 54, 186
Phenylpropanolamine, 99

Philosophy of continence, 123–124, 127, 153
Physical examination, 65–69
Polyuria, 53, 186
Pontine-mesencephalic gray matter, 8, 186
Postvoid residual (PVR), 55, 69, 73, 186
Precipitancy, 186
Pressure
  intraurethral, 5–6, 185
  intravesical, 2, 5–6, 9, 185
Pressure ulcers, 69, 186
Prevalence of urinary incontinence, 24–28, 187
Professional organizations, 190–191
Prolapse, 32–33, 55, 56, 187
Prompted voiding, 93–94, 162, 187
Propantheline bromide, 98
Prostate gland, 31, 187
  transurethral incision of (TUIP), 95
  transurethral resection of (TURP), 32, 95
Prostatectomy, 95
Prostatic hyperplasia, 11, 31–32, 182, 187
  assessment for, 65, 69
  incontinence after surgery for, 32, 95
  nursing care for man with, 133–141
  obstructive and irritative symptoms due to, 31, 32
Pseudoephedrine hydrochloride, 42, 99
Psychological care, 131–132, 137, 142–143, 148
Psychological impact of incontinence, 60–61, 86, 111–121
  to families, 118–119
  historical perspective on, 111–114
  to nursing staff, 119–120
  to older adult, 114–118
  questionnaires about, 117–118
Psychotropics, 187
Pubococcygeus muscle, 4, 87, 187
Pudendal nerve, 8
Pyridium, 102
Pyrilamine maleate, 42

R

Rectal examination, 69
Rectocele, 33, 69, 187
Research, 129–130
Resident Assessment Profile (RAP), 51, 102, 104, 187
Residual urine, 187

Resource allocation, 129
Restraint of patient, 102, 142
Review of systems, 56, 59–60

S

Sacral reflex center, 8, 187
Sanitation practices, 112
Sedative hypnotics, 40, 41, 104
Self-esteem, 86, 115, 132, 142
Self-management, 115, 116, 132, 162
Sensory impairments, 69, 101
Simon Foundation, 191
Skin care, 105, 128
Social support, 68
Society of Urologic Nurses and Associates, 191
Sphincter, 188
  urethral, 3, 183
Sphincter incompetence, 188
Spinal cord, 6–8
  sacral lesions of, 39
  suprasacral lesions of, 37–39
Stigma, 60
Subjective and objective manifestations of incontinence, 48
Supportive devices, 161–179
  absorbent bed protectors, 166
  bedpans, 170–172
  bedside commodes, 168
  benefits of, 161
  clothing, 174, 175
  congruence among behavioral therapies, outcomes, and, 162
  dampness detectors, 173–174
  different uses of, 161
  disposable absorbent products, 163–164
  environmental modifications, 166–167
  external collection devices for men, 172–173
  external collection devices for women, 173
  guidelines for use of, 178–179
  indwelling catheters, 174–178
  reusable briefs and products, 164–166
  timing devices, 173
  urinals for men, 168, 169
  urinals for women, 168–170
Surgery, 95–96

Sympathetic nervous system, 96, 188
Symphysis pubis, 188

T

Tabes dorsalis, 39
Terminology, 13–23, 181–189
Thioridazine hydrochloride, 42
Timing devices, 173
Toilet facilities, 43, 55, 102, 112–114, 143, 147–148, 166–167
Toileting
  patterned urge-response, 92–93
  scheduled, 92, 162, 187
Transurethral incision of prostate (TUIP), 95
Transurethral resection of prostate (TURP), 32, 95
Treatment of incontinence, 79–108
  in acute care setting, 107
  behavioral, 86–95
    behavioral modification, 91
    bladder training, 91–92
    electrical stimulation, 94–95
    habit training, 92–93
    pelvic floor training, 87–90
    prompted voiding, 93–94
    scheduled toileting, 92
  functional incontinence, 101–102
  guidelines for, 79, 86–87
  in home care setting, 107
  in long-term care setting, 104–107
  in man with benign prostatic hyperplasia, 133–138
  in older adult with functional incontinence secondary to dementia, 146–149
  in older man with transient incontinence secondary to delirium, 138, 142–143
  outcomes of, 105, 106, 162
  pharmacological, 96–100
  in postmenopausal woman with stress incontinence, 131–133
  supportive devices for, 161–179
  surgical, 95–96
  transient incontinence, 102–104
  voiding maneuvers, 100–101
Trigone of bladder, 2–3, 188

U

Upper neuron lesions, 188
Ureters, 1, 188

Urethra, 4–6, 188
  anatomic relationships of, 5, 7
  in men, 5, 6
    balloon dilation of, 95
    proximal, 187
  in women, 5, 69
    surgical repositioning of, 96
Urethral pressure profile, 188
Urethral sphincter, 3
  distal urethral sphincter mechanism, 183
Urethritis, 55, 56, 188
Urethrocele, 33, 69, 188
Urethrovesical angle, 33, 189
Urethrovesical junction, 33, 189
Urgency, 17, 65, 189
Urinals, 168–170, 189
Urinalysis, 69–70, 72–73
Urinary catheter, 182. *See also*
  Catheterization
  indwelling, 101, 107, 174–177
Urinary incontinence
  assessment of, 47–76, 80–85
  causes of, 25, 30–44, 80–85
  definition of, 13–15, 189
  established, 22, 183
  functional, 16, 48, 82–85, 101–102, 201
  overflow, 16, 20, 22, 48, 80, 82, 185
  pathophysiology of, 29
  patterns of, 22–23
  prevalence of, 24–28
  psychological impact of, 60–61, 86, 111–121
  reflex, 16, 17, 20
  stress, 15, 16, 34, 48, 80, 95–96, 188
  subjective and objective manifestations of, 48
  transient, 23, 30, 83–84, 102–104, 188
  treatment of, 79–108
  urge, 15–17, 18–19, 48, 81–82, 188

Urinary meatus, 189
Urinary retention, 42, 71, 92, 104, 189
Urinary tract infection (UTI), 35, 53–54, 102–103, 133, 149, 189
Urination, 189
Urine specimen collection, 54, 70
Urodynamic evaluation, 70–76
  assessment of urine flow, 70–73
  cystometrogram, 74–76
  pad test, 73
  postvoid residual, 73
Uroflowmeter, 71–73, 189
Urogenital system
  factors affecting continence, 31–35
  female, 32–33
  functional assessment of, 65
  male, 31

V

Vagina, 189
  examination of, 55–56, 69
  prolapse of anterior wall of, 33
Vaginal specula, 55
Vaginal weights, 90
Vaginitis, 55, 56, 189
Valsalva maneuver, 100
Vesica, 1, 189
Vision screening, 66
Voiding, 9, 189
  prompted, 93–94, 162, 187
Voiding maneuvers, 100–101
Voiding record, 62–63, 94

W

Weight reduction, 133
Wound, Ostomy, and Continence Nursing, 191

www.ingramcontent.com/pod-product-compliance
Ingram Content Group UK Ltd.
Pitfield, Milton Keynes, MK11 3LW, UK
UKHW021312180426
11947UKWH00015B/1185